PHYSICAL FITNESS, DIET AND EXERCISE

PHYSICAL ACTIVITY BEHAVIORS AND DETERMINANTS IN CHILDREN AND ADOLESCENTS

PHYSICAL FITNESS, DIET AND EXERCISE

Additional books in this series can be found on Nova's website under the Series tab.

Additional e-books in this series can be found on Nova's website under the e-book tab.

PHYSICAL FITNESS, DIET AND EXERCISE

PHYSICAL ACTIVITY BEHAVIORS AND DETERMINANTS IN CHILDREN AND ADOLESCENTS

ZAN GAO
AND
ZACHARY POPE
EDITORS

nova publishers
New York

Additional color graphics may be available in the e-book version of this book.

Library of Congress Cataloging-in-Publication Data

ISBN: 978-1-63483-635-7
Library of Congress Control Number: 2015948144

Published by Nova Science Publishers, Inc. † New York

CONTENTS

PREFACE

Children truly are the future. Each generation of youngsters represents a cohort of innovators with a plethora of unique talents rooted in the resources available to them during their formative years. For instance, the technology available to the current generation of youngsters was once unimaginable two decades ago. This technology allows today's youth to not only acquire, but produce knowledge faster than ever before—a fact which provides the opportunity for intrepid individuals with big ideas to make a meaningful impact in the world. However, what if current and future generations are too unhealthy to fully carry out or pursue their dreams? That same technology that provides such power to the current generation of youth has also created an obesogenic environment which makes engaging in copious amounts of sedentary activities all too easy for children.

Ever the optimists, however, the editors of this book believe that the current poor health of youth is not beyond intervention—especially if the individual(s) intervening to promote healthier behaviors among youth are doing so from a solid, empirical base. In this accord, the editors wanted to offer information for researchers and practitioners set on promoting improved health among youth through well designed theory-based physical activity interventions. In order to achieve this mission, it was clear the contributors to this book needed to be diverse in their expertise. As such, contributors to this book include individuals from the fields of physical education to physical activity epidemiology with decades of combined experience in the implementation of physical activity interventions among youth. The impetus for this book was simple in that through the provision of high quality original research, researchers in the fields of physical education, health education, physical activity epidemiology, as well as community health, might be able to use the theory-driven physical activity intervention strategies detailed within the included chapters to promote more healthful behaviors among youth. Implementing these physical activity intervention strategies might just provide youth the opportunity to grow up happy and healthy while also ensuring that anything this talented generation of children set their mind to, they can achieve. With this goal in mind, below are a number of characteristics the reader might expect to find within the current book:

- A compilation of seven original empirical research articles examining the use of theoretically-driven physical activity interventions in the promotion of youth physical activity and health, as well as a final chapter devoted to the review of correlates and determinants of physical activity outcomes among youth.
- Application of several widely used theoretical frameworks in the research projects including social ecologic model, protection motivation theory, self-efficacy theory, situational interest theory, and competence motivation theory.
- Targeting a variety of youth populations in the aforementioned projects including elementary school children, young adolescents, and older adolescents.
- Theoretical and practical implications of findings as they relate to promotion of youth's physical activity participation in multiple contexts including various school- and community-based settings.
- Clear and easy-to-follow writing structure, which allows researchers and practitioners to implement the interventions discussed among their own youth population of interest.

Hopefully, the individual reading this book believes the above characteristics to be true as the editors and contributors alike wanted to produce a book which demonstrated scientific rigor while also being practical enough that the concepts and ideas introduced could be transferred into the real-world contexts. That being said, we ask that you go forth and enjoy the information presented in the book and hope that, by doing so, you are able to make a significant impact in the lives of the youth you work with while providing them the greatest opportunity to be happy, healthy, and successful.

In: Physical Activity Behaviors …
Editors: Zan Gao and Zachary Pope
ISBN: 978-1-63483-635-7

Chapter 1

ADOLESCENT GIRLS' PHYSICAL ACTIVITY DETERMINANTS AND PHYSICAL ACTIVITY PARTICIPATION: AN APPLICATION OF THE SOCIAL ECOLOGICAL MODEL

Huiping Sheng[1], Zachary Pope[2] and Zan Gao[2,*]
[1]WellCare Health Plans Inc., Tampa, FL, US
[2]University of Minnesota-Twin Cities, Minneapolis, MN, US

ABSTRACT

Literature suggests adolescent girls' physical activity levels vary by social and individual factors. Most research, however, has focused on individual factors with linear relationship analyses. This study utilized the Social Ecological Model and structural equation modeling to identify determinants of adolescent girls' physical activity levels. Participants were 217 middle school girls (Mean age = 12) in grades 6-8 from six schools in New Mexico, U.S. in 2007. Girls' physical activity determinants were measured subjectively by three questionnaires, while physical activity was assessed objectively by pedometers. Results indicated socioeconomic status was a significant contributor to girls' physical activity levels (steps/minute), predicting girls' physical activity through the mediating factor of sedentary habits. Additionally, the effect

[*] Corresponding Author address: 207 Cooke Hall, 1900 University Ave. SE, Minneapolis, MN, 55455; Email: gaoz@umn.edu.

of socioeconomic status was mediated by self-efficacy, which was further mediated by sedentary habits with socioeconomic status also found to be a precursor of both the aforementioned variables. Notably, girls' self-efficacy had a negative association with sedentary habits (r = - 0.26). Finally, parents' supportive attitude towards their daughters' physical activity participation was positively correlated with their daughters' sports team participation (r = 0.36). Findings support literature indicating socioeconomic status to be a predictor of adolescent physical activity. Further, the results suggest structured physical activity interventions which increase the physical activity self-efficacy of adolescent girls are needed.

Keywords: physical activity levels, self-efficacy, socioeconomic status, youth physical activity promotion model

INTRODUCTION

The overweight and obesity crisis among adolescents is of concern in the U.S. with low physical activity levels seen as a major contributing factor. The American College of Sports Medicine recommends adolescents engage in 60 minutes of daily physical activity (Pescatello, Arena, Riebe, & Thompson, 2013). Unfortunately, research indicates 20% to 50% of adolescents engage in insufficient physical activity and 6% to 12% do not perform any moderate or vigorous physical activity at all (Corbin, Pangrazi, & Le Masurier, 2004). It is, therefore, important to understand the underlying determinants of physical activity participation among adolescents.

Resulting from the need to understand physical activity determinants in adolescents, researchers have hypothesized what factors contribute to the profile of physically active youth. Castelli and Erwin (2007) listed many contextual and individual factors contributing to the profile of physically active youth: regular participation in physical education and youth sports, time spent outdoors, participatory support from parents/siblings, motor skill proficiency and physical fitness. Moreover, Dennis (2012) indicated that children do not view exercise as a way to remain fit, instead valuing the psychological rewards of social interaction, feelings of personal success, and enjoyment. These rewards, in turn, influence children's self-efficacy of which is a vital component of physical activity behavior (Bandura, 1977a, 1977b). Thus, the school, home, and community environments, as well as children's self-efficacy, each play an important role in promoting physical activity among children.

Increasing children's physical activity levels through intervention strategies associated with the aforementioned contexts/psychosocial variables necessitates a thorough understanding of physical activity determinants in adolescents. This study was designed to investigate adolescent girls' physical activity determinants and effects of these determinants on physical activity levels utilizing the framework of the Social Ecological Model (Bronfenbrenner, 1979). Within this theoretical framework, Welk (1999; see Figure 1) proposed the Youth Physical Activity Promotion Model consisting of: (1) reinforcement from family, peers, or coaches; (2) individual factors like beliefs, attitudes, or self-efficacy; (3) demographics; and (4) students' enabling factors such as fitness level, motor skills, and access to physical activity environments. This model provides a theoretical framework suggesting children's physical activity is influenced by multiple contextual and individual factors, but it has seldom been quantified within the literature to further identify the relationship among these multiple factors. In many previous studies, only linear model analyses of these relationships have been conducted, which may not be sufficient in addressing the complexity of adolescents' physical activity environments (Malouf & Schiller, 1995). Specifically, research suggests many environmental (e.g., social support for physical activity, access to physical activity facilities), cultural (e.g., family physical activity beliefs, cultural physical activity preferences), and individual factors (e.g., self-efficacy, outcome expectancy) may present roadblocks for children's physical activity participation (Biddle, Whitehead, O'Donovan, & Nevill, 2005; Molnar, Gortmaker, Bull, & Buka, 2004; Saelens, Sallis, Biack, & Chen, 2003; Wu, Pender, & Noureddine, 2003; Zlot, Librett, Buchner, & Schmid, 2006), indicating more complex analyses of physical activity determinants, such as the social ecological model, need to take place.

Further, research supports the need to investigate the physical activity determinants of adolescent girls and ethnic minorities. For example, Riddoch and colleagues (2004) found that regardless of age, boys (9-15 years-old) were more active than girls; a result which reached significance at age 15. Moreover, the decline in adolescent girls' physical activity levels was steeper as a function of increasing age compared to boys. Regarding the effect of ethnicity on physical activity, Allen and associates (2007) indicated that the physical activity levels of Asian and Latino 12-17 years-old children to be significantly lower than that of non-Hispanic whites. These findings are of concern as children and adolescents who live less physically active lifestyles are subject to poorer long-term health than children and adolescents who are more physically active (Dohle & Wansink, 2013; Reilly & Kelly, 2011).

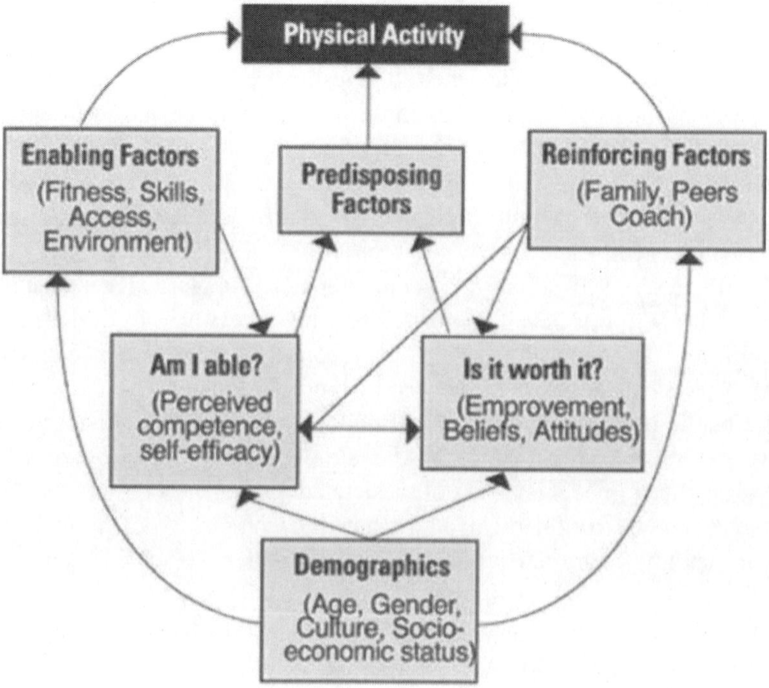

Figure 1. A Conceptual Diagram of the Youth Physical Activity Promotion Model (Welk, 1999).

Given that scholars posit multiple levels of physical activity determinants influence physical activity participation (see Sallis et al., 2006), a need exists to examine adolescent girls' physical activity determinants and participation as it pertains to the multiple factors within the Social Ecological Model. Further, as previously mentioned, these studies need to take place within an ethnically diverse population. The current research was conducted in several ethnically diverse New Mexico schools wherein 30% of the children are at risk of becoming or are currently overweight (New Mexico Department of Health, 2004) with the aim of examining the predictive strengths of adolescent girls' physical activity determinants on objectively-measured physical activity levels using structural equation modelling. This investigation was guided by the following two research questions: (1) Which determinants were related to adolescent girls' physical activity levels? and (2) To what magnitude did these determinants predict adolescent girls' physical activity levels? The findings may provide empirical evidence to promote adolescent girls' physical activity levels, and offer implications to maximize the function of certain determinants within the school, family, and communities.

METHODS

Participants

A convenience sample of 389 participants from six schools in Albuquerque, New Mexico, voluntarily agreed to participate in this cross-sectional study. Of the original sample, some girls declined to participate in the study, dropped out, or provided invalid data resulting in a final sample of 217 girls and their parents or guardians (57% retention). The final sample included 81 sixth (37.3%), 70 seventh (32.3%), and 66 eighth (30.4%) grade girls, ranging in age from 10 to 13 ($Mean_{age}$ = 12 years). More than half (129, 59.4%) of the household incomes were above $50,001/year which was higher than the median New Mexico household income of $42,760 for 2006-2007 (U.S. Census Bureau, 2004). The education distribution was: 18%, 23%, 22.6%, 17.1%, and 19.4% for graduate, bachelor, professional college, high school, and lower than high school, respectively, representing 83.8% mothers, 14.7% of fathers, and 1.5% of others who took the survey. Race/ethnicity of the sample was as follows: 50.7% Hispanic-American, 29.0% Caucasian, 15.2% African American, 5.1% American Indian and others (see Table 1).

Instruments

One biographical information sheet, assent and consent forms, three survey documents, and one pedometer instrument for each participant were used in this study. These assessments were utilized to assess adolescent girls' physical activity determinants and physical activity levels.

State and Local Middle School Youth Risk Behavior Survey (SLMSYRBS) for Children. The State and Local Middle School Youth Risk Behavior Survey is a modified instrument of the 2007 Middle School Youth Risk Behavior Survey and has acceptable reliability and validity of kappa 61%-100% (Centers for Disease Control and Prevention, 2003, 2004). The questionnaire consists of 14 multiple choice questions regarding demographic information and physical activity behavior. For example, the girls were asked: “On how many of the past seven days did you participate with your parents in physical activity for at least 30 minutes, such as fast walking, slow bicycling, skating, exercising in the park?” The response options were 0 to 7 days.

Table 1. Demographic Information of Study Students

	School 1	*School 2*	*School 3*	*School 4*	*School 5*	*School 6*	*total*	*%*
# of subjects	51	14	55	37	32	28	217	
Age (Y) *	12	11	12	12	12	12	12	
Grade								
6	22	13	27	14	0	5	81	37.3
7	18	1	14	10	18	9	70	32.3
8	11	0	14	13	14	14	66	30.4
Ethnicity								
Caucasian	23	6	7	21	4	2	63	29.0
Hispanic (a)	26	6	41	10	25	2	110	50.7
AA*	2	2	6	2	1	22	33	15.2
AI** and others	0	0	1	4	2	2	11	5.1

Note: *: African American, **: American Indian.

Self-Efficacy for Children. Adolescent girls' physical activity self-efficacy was assessed via a questionnaire organized into two categories of short response items adapted from the *Guide for Constructing Self-efficacy Scales* (Bandura, 2006). All items were rated on 100% confidence scales from “0” for “*cannot do at all*” to “100” for “*highly certain can do*.” The questionnaire has shown high internal reliability (*Cronbach's alpha=.92*). The first category, self-efficacy to regulate exercise, had 18 short response questions. One example was “I am confident in my ability (0-100) to perform regular exercise 3 or more times a week when I have other interesting things to do.” The mean scores of the 18 items gave an indication of the magnitude of a girl's self-efficacy to perform the exercise routine regularly. Means for the 8-item second category gave an indication of the magnitude of a girl's self-efficacy about leisure time skills and extracurricular activities. The average score of the two categories of self-efficacy was used to represent girls' physical activity self-efficacy.

Youth Media Campaign Longitudinal Survey for Parents. The Youth Media Campaign Longitudinal Survey for Parents is an interviewer-administered telephone survey designed to evaluate the effects of the U.S. Centers for Disease Control and Prevention's VERB campaign (Huhman, Heitzier, & Wong, 2004). Acceptable reliability for the estimation of free-time activity and total weekly physical activity has been seen with this measure (intraclass correlation = 0.60 and intraclass correlation = 0.60, respectively) (Huhman, Heitzier, & Wong, 2004). This survey assessed organized and free-time physical activity performed outside of school and was adaptable to populations of interest (Centers for Disease Control and Prevention, 2003; Welk et al., 2007).

In this study, the Youth Media Campaign Longitudinal Survey was converted from a telephone survey to a self-administered 22-item survey for participating parents consisting of information concerning parents/legal guardians' demographic information, physical activity, attitude towards their child's physical activity, confidence in being able to influence their child's physical activity, their physical activity support for their child, and their child's physical activity behavior.

Physical Activity Levels. To assess girls' physical activity levels, W4L Neo II pedometers (Walk4Life Inc., Oswego, IL) were used to count daily steps and physical activity duration in minutes for four consecutive school days. W4L pedometers are valid and reliable in measuring ambulatory physical activity (Bassett et al., 2000; Bassett & Strath, 2002; Crouter, Schneider, Karabulut, & Bassett, 2003; Graser, Pangrazi, & Vincent, 2007; Schneider, Crouter, & Bassett, 2004; Schneider, Crouter, Lukajic, & Bassett, 2003). A mean total of 22 hours of physical activity monitoring was conducted on each girl over the course of four consecutive school days. The dependent variable was steps per minute. During the data collection, 10 (20%) pedometers were lost by the participants.

Procedures

This study was approved by the Human Subject Institutional Review Board at the University of New Mexico. Assent was obtained from each participating girl while consent was obtained from parents/legal guardians. The principal investigator was responsible for collecting all the physical activity and self-reported physical activity determinants data. The three questionnaires and assent/consent forms were distributed to potential participants and their parents/legal guardians in one large envelope packet at the beginning of the data collection period at each school. The assent and consent forms were obtained prior to the collection of the questionnaires, after which the principal investigator collected the physical activity data using the pedometers and administered the surveys to the girls and their parents.

Data Analyses

In line with the study purpose, this investigation was a multivariate, three-level social ecological based modeling study (see Figure 2) based on the Welk Youth Physical Activity Promotion Model (Welk, 1999). The dependent variable was student's physical activity levels as assessed by steps per minute. The independent variables were demographic factors (age, ethnicity, social-economic status), environmental factors [family, school, community], and girls' physical activity self-efficacy).

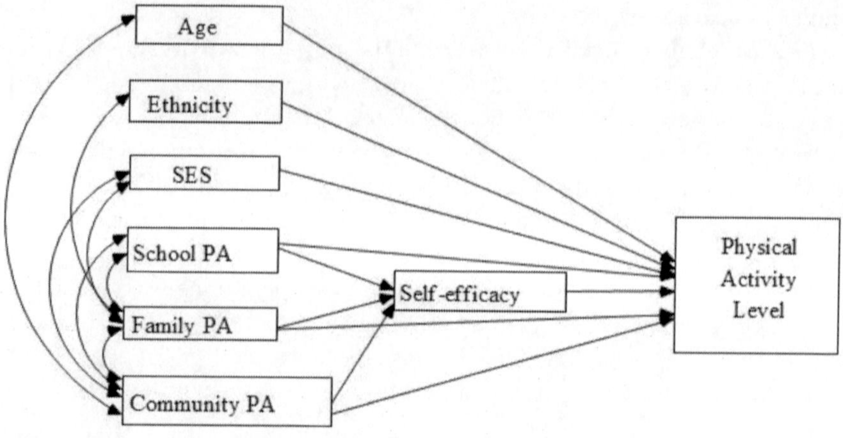

Figure 2. Adolescent Girl's Physical Activiry Determinants.

Data were analyzed through SPSS 15.0 (SPSS, Inc., Chicago, IL) and AMOS (Analysis of Moment Structures) 15.0 (SPSS, Inc., Chicago, IL) as follows: 1) the internal consistency of the self-reported data was confirmed; 2) Pearson correlations were calculated between independent variables to reveal associations between the study variables; and 3) a series of path analyses were employed using AMOS, to test the interceding effects of the mediating variable, self-efficacy, within the hypothesized model. The model fit was then assessed based on the following indices: chi-square root (χ^2), mean square root error of approximation (RMSEA), and the comparative fit index (CFI). The model which best fit the data was identified by examining significant correlations and changing some theoretical assumptions related to the model. This analytical process helped the researchers discern which variables determined adolescent girls' physical activity levels and to what degree each variable predicts the middle school girls' physical activity levels.

RESULTS

Cronbach alpha coefficients for the latent variables were as follows: 0.62 for environment, 0.53 for family physical activity, 0.86 for sports team participation, 0.89 for parents' attitude, 0.60 for habits, 0.58 for socioeconomic status, and 0.92 for self-efficacy. Thus, the results indicated that internal consistency met the requirements for model fit. Three indices were then used to test the fit of the final model: the chi-square ratio, CFI and RMSEA were selected as they are least affected by sample size (Fan, Thompson, & Wang, 1999).

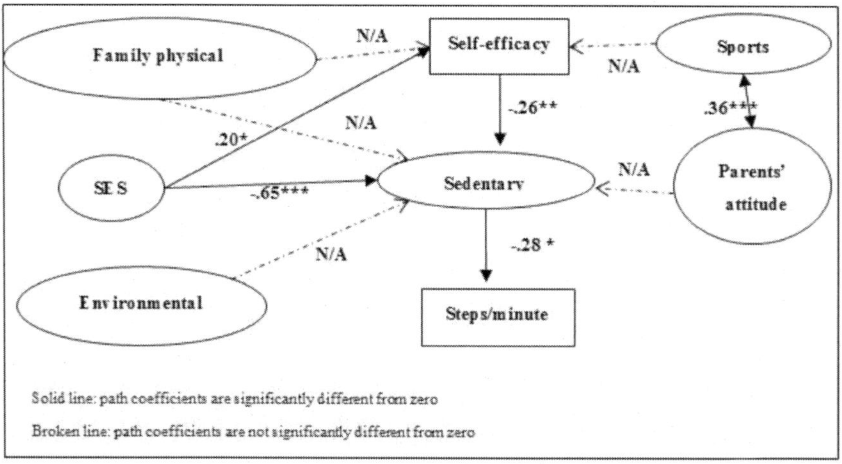

Note: *** *p-val* < .001; ** *p-val* < .01; * *p-val* < .05; [1]fixed at 1 in non-standardized solution. The sign (+, -) indicated the positive (+) or negative (-) relationship between vatiables.

Figure 3. Social Ecological Model to Predict Adolescent Girl's Physical Activity Levels.

The above three fit indices of models were 2.50; 1; and 0.08. Accordingly, the results showed that the social ecological model met the acceptable model fit requirements and, thus, the model could be used to test the hypothesis-based model.

Figure 3 shows the model obtained from AMOS 15.0 program as a parsimonious model demonstrating the social ecological determinants predicting adolescent girls' physical activity levels. Since the path coefficients are standardized regression weight, the contributions of different latent variables can be compared directly from the absolute coefficient value. As demonstrated in Figure 3, socioeconomic status significantly contributed to girls' physical activity levels (i.e., steps per minute). Specifically, socioeconomic status was positively associated with girls' physical activity self-efficacy ($r = .20$), but negatively associated with sedentary habits ($r =- 0.65$). Second, socioeconomic status indirectly predicted girls' physical activity levels via the mediating factor of sedentary habits. Further, as a determinant of girls' physical activity levels, socioeconomic status was mediated by self-efficacy, which was further mediated by sedentary habits. Thus, we concluded that socioeconomic status was a precursor to self-efficacy and sedentary habits, which in turn predicted girls' physical activity levels. Additionally, parents' supportive attitude toward their daughters' physical activity participation was positively correlated with girls' sports team participation experience ($r = 0.36$). Finally, girls' self-efficacy negatively predicted sedentary habits ($r =- 0.26$) while sedentary habits were negatively associated with physical activity ($r =- 0.28$). Within the model, the demographic, environmental factors, and girls' self-efficacy directly influenced their physical activity levels. The demographic and environmental factors also influenced girls' self-efficacy, acting as a possible mediator between the demographic/environmental factors, and physical activity levels.

Discussion

The present study suggests adolescent girls' physical activity levels were strongly predicted by the social factor of family socioeconomic status as well as the individual factors of physical activity self-efficacy and personal sedentary habits such as watching television/playing video games. Studies regarding socioeconomic status have indicated that higher socioeconomic status was associated with increased physical activity among children. Specifically, research indicates wealthier school districts offer more physical activity/sport opportunities for girls in addition to middle- and upper- class parents being better able to support their daughters' physical activity (Biddle et al., 2005; Gordon-Larsen, Adair, & Popkin, 2002; Lioret, Touvier, Lafay, Volatier, & Maire, 2008; Richmond, Field, & Rich, 2007). Results of the current study appear to corroborate results of previous literature indicating socioeconomic status to be a major physical activity determinant.

Regarding the current findings that adolescent girls' physical activity was significantly predicted by physical activity self-efficacy, this finding is also aligned with previous literature. Studies of the relationship between self-efficacy and physical activity have demonstrated self-efficacy to be predictive of physical activity behavior in youth (See Annesi, 2006; Hausenblas, Nigg, Downs, Fleming, & Connaughton, 2002) and that structured intervention programs can promote enhanced self-efficacy and increased physical activity levels (Annesi, Faigenbaum, & Westcott, 2010). As for the findings regarding the inverse relationship between girls' sedentary habits and physical activity, Malina (2008) suggests that adolescent girls' maturational status during puberty may result in lower self-esteem and changes in the interests of girls which may not be aligned with physical activity. As such, one might hypothesize the new interests of adolescent girls to be sedentary activities based on the results of the current study. Caution should be taken, however, when making this conclusion as research has shown sedentary habits do not necessarily displace physical activity engagement (Vandewater, Bickham, & Lee, 2006). Thus, more research on the relationship of adolescent girls' sedentary habits and physical activity is advised.

The present study is one of a growing number of investigations completed regarding how the multiple factors of the social ecological model might influence physical activity levels (Stevens et al., 2005; Webber et al., 2008). Findings from the current study indicate factors such as the family's physical activity, family environment, sports team participation, and parents' attitudes toward physical activity predicted, to some degree, adolescent girls' physical activity levels when entered into the model individually. Yet, results make clear that socioeconomic status, physical activity self-efficacy, and sedentary habits are the most significant predictors of physical activity overall. As a result of such findings, practical implications can be recommended which improve the alignment of the preceding factors with greater physical activity participation among adolescent girls.

First, school administrators and educators should devote their efforts toward promoting girls' physical activity participation by providing gender neutral activities which interest both boys and girls and, perhaps, provide same-sex physical education options. Second, given that adolescent girls of lower socioeconomic status are at greater risk of lower physical activity than higher socioeconomic status adolescent girls, efforts to promote physical activity participation among this high-risk population is needed in the form of physical education interventions and after school programs. Failure to do so might cause the socioeconomic status-related health disparities to widen.

One manner to attenuate socioeconomic status disparities is to provide more community-based physical activity opportunities in low socioeconomic status districts with funding for more public exercise facilities, easier access to parks or walking trails, and free after-school programs in community centers. Moreover, community organizers within these communities can promote family physical activity programs with the objective to enhance parents' positive attitude towards their daughters' physical activity. Finally, enhancing girls' self-efficacy in physical education classes can increase their physical activity levels. Lastly, from physical education teacher education to K-12 physical education curriculum design, effective strategies should be sought to enhance children's self-efficacy toward physical activity participation.

Strengths of this study include the study's purposeful sampling of adolescent girls at risk for lower physical activity participation and overweight/obesity in addition to the examination of the factors affecting physical activity participation via socioeconomic status with an analysis of these factors using structural equation modelling. Despite these strengths, the current study has limitations worth noting. To begin, the study represents data collected in 2007. Given the changes to adolescents' physical activity environment brought about by Health People 2010 and 2020 (U.S. Department for Health and Human Services, 2005), it is possible that the factors associated with adolescent girls' physical activity participation are different in the present day. It is, therefore, recommended that future research continue to investigate the factors associated with the physical activity participation of adolescent girls utilizing the tenets of social ecological model. A second limitation is the use of a relatively small sample from one geographic location of which decreases the generalizability of the study's findings. It is suggested that future research include a larger number of adolescent girls from widespread locations across the U.S. Finally, although pilot testing was completed for the current study, the surveys used for the assessment of physical activity determinants had to be modified slightly which could be seen as a potential limitation of the current investigation. In this accord, future studies may want to use questionnaires specifically developed for administration to adolescent girls which may have been developed in the seven years since the conclusion of this study.

CONCLUSION

The findings of this study suggest that many physical activity determinants work together in a true social ecological environment to predict adolescent girls' physical activity levels. The results, therefore, indicate that a holistic approach for adolescent girls' overall well-being is a priority in the promotion of increased physical activity in this population. Simply put, it is critical to motivate adolescent girls to value physical activity for health benefits.

REFERENCES

Allen, M., Elliott, M., Morales, L., Diamant, A., Hambarsoomian, K., & Schuster, M. (2007). Adolescent participation in preventitive health behaviors, physical activity, and nutrition: Differences across immigrant generations for Asians and Latinos compared with Whites. *American Journal of Public Health, 97*(2), 337-343.

Annesi, J. (2006). Relations of physical self-concept and self-efficacy with frequency of voluntary physical activity in preadolescents: Implications for after-school care programing. *Journal of Psychosomatic Research, 61*, 515-520.

Annesi, J., Faigenbaum, A., & Westcott, W. (2010). Relations of transtheoretical model stage, self-efficacy, and voluntary physical activity in African American preadolescents. *Research Quarterly for Exercise and Sport, 81*(2), 239-244.

Bandura, A. (1977a). Self-efficacy: Toward a unifying theory of behavioral change. *Psychological Review, 84,* 191-215.

Bandura, A. (1977b). *Social learning theory.* Englewood Cliffs, NJ: Prentice Hall.

Bandura, A. (2006). Guide for constructing self-efficacy scales (pp. 307-337). In Pajares, F, Urdan, T eds. *Self-Efficacy Beliefs of Adolescents.* Greenwich, CT: Information Age Publishing.

Bassett, D.R., Ainsworth, B.E., Swartz, A.M., Strath, S.J., O'Brien, W.L., & King, G.A. (2000). Validity of four motions sensors in measuring moderate intensity physical activity. *Medicine & Science in Sport & Exercise, 32*(S9), S471-S480.

Bassett, D.R., & Strath, S.J. (2002). Use of pedometers to assess physical activity (pp. 163-177). In Gregory Welk (Ed.). *Physical Activity Assessments for Health-Related Research.* Champaign, IL: Human Kinetics.

Biddle, S.J.H., Whitehead, S.H., O'Donovan, T.M., & Nevill, M.E. (2005). Correlates of participation in physical activity for adolescent girls: A systematic literature review of recent literature. *Journal of Physical Activity and Health, 2*(4), 423-434.

Bronfenbrenner, U. (1979). *The Ecology of Human Development: Experiments by Nature and Design.* Cambridge, MA: Harvard University Press.

Castelli, D.M. & Erwin, E.H. (2007). Chapter 4: A comparison of personal attributes and experiences among physically active and inactive children. *Journal of Teaching in Physical Education, 26,* 375-389.

Centers for Disease Control and Prevention. (2003). Physical activity level. *Morbidity & Mortality Weekly Report, 52*(33), 785-788.

Centers for Disease Control and Prevention. (2004) Participation in high school. *Morbidity & Mortality Weekly Report, 53*(36), 844-847.

Corbin, CB., Pangrazi, PR., & Le Masurier, C.G. (2004). Physical activity for children: Current patterns and guidelines. *President's Council on Physical Fitness and Sports Research Digest, 5*(2), 1-8.

Crouter, S.E., Schneider, P.L., Karabulut, M., & Bassett, D.R. (2003). Validity of ten electronic pedometers for measuring distance walked. *Medicine & Science in Sport & Exercise, 35*(5), S283.

Dennis, C. (2012). Kids, kids, kids. Retrieved from http://scwfitness.com/index.php?story=1079&fmt=1

Dohle, S., & Wansink, B. (2013). Fit in 50 years: Participation in high school sports best predicts one's physical activity after age 70. *BMC Public Health, 13*(1100). Retrieved from: http://www.biomedcentral.com/1471-2458/13/1100

Fan, X., Thompson, B., & Wang. L. (1999). The effects of sample size, estimation methods, and model specification on SEM fit indices. *Structural Equation Modeling, 6*, 56-83.

Gordon-Larsen, P., Adair, L.S., & Popkin, B.M. (2002). Ethnic differences in physical activity and inactivity patterns and overweight status. *Obesity Research & Clinical Practice, 10*(3), 141-149.

Graser, S.V., Pangrazi, R.P., & Vincent, J.W. (2007). Effects of placement, attachment, and weight classification on pedometer accuracy. *Journal of Physical Activity and Health, 4*, 359-369.

Hausenblas, H., Nigg, C., Downs, D., Fleming, D., & Connaughton, D. (2002). Perceptions of exercise stages, barrier self-efficacy, and decisional balance for middle-level school students. *Journal of Early Adolescence, 22*(4), 436-454.

Huhman, M., Heitzier, C., & Wong, F. (2004). The VERB campaign logic model: a tool for planning and evaluation. *Preventing Chronic Disease*. Retrieved from http://www.cdc.gov/pcd/issues2004/toc.htm.

Lioret, S., Touvier, M., Lafay, L., Volatier, J.L., & Maire, B. (2008). Are eating occasions and their energy content related to child overweight and socioeconomic status? *Obesity, 16*(11), 2518-2523.

Malina, R. (2008). Biocultural factors in developing physical activity levels (pp. 141-167). In Alan Smith & Stuart Biddle (Eds.). *Youth Physical Activity and Sedentary Behavior: Challenges and Solutions*. Champaign, IL: Human Kinetics.

Molnar, B.E., Gortmaker, S.L., Bull, F.C., & Buka, S.L. (2004). Health promoting community design unsafe to play? Neighborhood disorder and lack of safety predict reduced physical activity among urban children and adolescents. *American Journal of Health Promotion, 18*(5), 378–386.

Malouf, D.B. & Schiller, E.P. (1995). Practice and research in special education. *Except Children, 61,* 414-424.

New Mexico Department of Health. (2004). New Mexico Youth Risk and Resiliency Survey. Report of State Results.

Pescatello, L., Arena, R., Riebe, D., & Thompson, P. (2013). *ACSM's Guidelines for Exercise Testing and Prescription* (9th ed.). Baltimore, MD: Lippincott Williams & Wilkins.

Reilly, J., & Kelly, J. (2011) Long-term impact of overweight and obesity in childhood and adolescence on morbidity and premature mortality in adulthood: Systematic review. *International Journal of Obesity, 35,* 891-898.

Richmond, T.K., Field, A.E., & Rich, M. (2007). Can neighborhoods explain racial/ethnic differences in adolescent inactivity? *International Journal of Pediatric Obesity, 2*(4), 202-210.

Riddoch, C., Andersen, L., Wedderkopp, N., Harro, M., Klasson-Heggebo, L., Sardinha, L.,… & Ekelund, U. (2004). Physical activity levels and patterns of 9- and 15-yr-old European children. *Medicine & Science in Sport & Exercise, 36*(1), 86-92.

Sallis, F.J., Cervero, B.R., Ascher, W., Henderson, A.K., Kraft, K.M., & Kerr, J. (2006). An ecological approach to creating active living communities. *Annual Review of Public Health, 27,* 297-322.

Saelens, B.T., Sallis, J.F., Biack, J.B., & Chen, D. (2003). Neighborhood-based differences in physical activity: An environment scale evaluation. *American Journal of Public Health, 93*(9), 1552-1558.

Schneider, P.L., Crouter, S.E., & Bassett, D.R. (2004). Pedometer measures of free-living physical activity: Comparison of 13 models. *Medicine & Science in Sport & Exercise, 36*(2), 331-335.

Schneider, P.L., Crouter, S.E., Lukajic, O., & Bassett, D.R. (2003). Accuracy and reliability of 10 pedometers for measuring steps over a 400-m walk. *Medicine & Science in Sport & Exercise, 35*(10), 1779-1784.

Stevens, J., Murray, D.M., Catellier, D.J., Hannan, P.J., Lytele, L.A., Elder, J.P.,...Webber, L.S. (2005). Design of the Trial of Activity in Adolescent Girls (TAAG). *Contemporary Clinical Trials*, *25*, 223-233.

U.S. Census Bureau. (2004). Current Population Survey, 2005 to 2008 Annual Social and Economic Supplements. Retrieved from http://search.census.gov/search?q=Current+Population+Survey&entqr=0&ud=1&output=xml_no_dtd&oe=UTF-8&ie=UTF-8&client=default_frontend&proxystyle sheet=default_frontend&site=census

USDHHS. (2005). *Healthy People 2010 and Steps to a HealthierUS: Leading Prevention.* Retrieved from http://www.healthypeople.gov/2010/Implementation/slides/HP_Steps_03262004.ppt

Vandewater, E., Bickham, D., & Lee, J. (2006). Time well spent? Relating television use to children's free-time activities. *Pediatrics*, *117*(2), e181-e191.

Webber, L.S., Catellier, D.J., Lytle, L.A., Murray, D.M., Pratt, C.A., Young, D.R.,...Pate, R.R. (2008). Promoting physical activity in middle school girls: Trial of Activity for Adolescent Girls. *American Journal of Preventive Medicine, 34*(3), 173-184..

Welk, G.J. (1999). The youth physical activity promotion model: A conceptual bridge between theory and practice. *Quest*, *51,* 5-23.

Welk, G.J., Wickel, E., Peterson, M., Heitzier, C.D., Fulton, J.E., & Potter, L.D. (2007). Reliability and validity of questions on the Youth Media Campaign Longitudinal Survey. *Medicine & Science in Sport & Exercise, 39*(4), 612-621.

Wu, T.Y., Pender, N., & Noureddine, S. (2003). Gender differences in the psychosocial and cognitive correlates of physical activity among Taiwanese adolescents: A structural equation modeling approach. *International Journal of Behavioral Medicine, 10*(2), 93-105.

Zlot, A.I., Librett, J., Buchner, D., & Schmid, T. (2006). Environmental, transportation, social, and time barriers to physical activity. *Journal of Physical Activity and Health, 3,*15-21.

In: Physical Activity Behaviors …
Editors: Zan Gao and Zachary Pope
ISBN: 978-1-63483-635-7

Chapter 2

Adolescent Girls' Physical Activity Levels in New Mexico: Status, Determinants, and Measurement Issues

Huiping Sheng[1], Zachary Pope[2] and Zan Gao[2,*]
[1]WellCare Health Plans Inc., Tampa, FL, US
[2]University of Minnesota-Twin Cities, Minneapolis, MN, US

Abstract

Adolescent girls of ethnic minorities are at increased risk of chronic diseases (e.g., Type 2 diabetes, obesity) partially resulting from low levels of physical activity. As such, a concerted effort needs to be made to understand the relevant physical activity determinants which might be present in these populations as doing so will allow for the implementation of more successful physical activity interventions. The purpose of this study was to investigate the current status and determinants of physical activity in an ethnically diverse sample of adolescent girls in New Mexico in addition to examining potential issues related to physical activity measurement within this population. A total of 217 adolescent girls (81 sixth, 70 seventh, and 66 eighth grade students; $Mean_{age}$ = 12 years) participated in this study. The race/ethnicity characteristics of the

* Corresponding Author address: 207 Cooke Hall, 1900 University Ave. SE, Minneapolis, MN, 55455 Email: gaoz@umn.edu.

sample were as follows: 50.7% Hispanic-American, 29.0% Caucasian, 15.2% African American, and 5.1% American Indian and others. Adolescent girls and their parents/guardians responded to a battery of questionnaires assessing daily physical activity levels and determinants. Further, adolescent girls' objective daily physical activity levels were measured by W4L Neo II pedometers for four consecutive days. The data analyses yielded the following findings: 1) On average, New Mexico adolescent girls' physical activity levels met the recommended duration for health promotion (mean daily physical activity time = 75.44 minutes); 2) Socioeconomic status emerged as the major physical activity determinant and mediated the effect of ethnicity on physical activity; 3) girls had moderate levels of physical activity self-efficacy for regular physical activity participation (mean = 51.64, standard deviation = 21.56). Further analysis revealed only one ethnic difference in self-efficacy wherein African American girls had significantly higher self-efficacy for learning dance skills than White girls (mean difference: 24.11, $p = 0.01$). Regarding the determinants of adolescent girls' physical activity self-efficacy, grade level was not found to be a significant predictor ($p = 0.29$) but age ($p = 0.06$) and ethnicity ($p = 0.01$) demonstrated marginally significantly and positive relationships with adolescent girls' physical activity self-efficacy, respectively; and 4) Girls' self-reported physical activity levels accurately reflected the objective, pedometer-determined moderate intensity physical activity. Results indicate socioeconomic status to be the largest mediator of ethnicity-related differences in physical activity participation among adolescent girls. Further, the findings also suggest that self-efficacy for learning certain types of physical activities was higher in some ethnic groups than in other ethnic groups (e.g., high self-efficacy for learning dance in African American girls). Therefore, physical activity interventions with adolescent girls should concentrate on establishing programs within low socioeconomic status schools or community centers which tailor curriculum to the physical activity preferences of the ethnic group being served.

Keywords: physical activity, ethnicity, self-efficacy

INTRODUCTION

Low physical activity in adolescence has been associated with a dramatic increase in the prevalence of obesity and onset of cardiovascular disease risk factors (Hedley et al., 2004). Regular participation in physical activity as an adolescent is critical to not only reduce the incidence of overweight, diabetes and other chronic health diseases in this population, but to also help adolescents develop and maintain the skills needed to engage in healthy lifestyle behaviors (Ballard et al., 2005). Schools are often indicated as venues wherein adolescent physical activity can be promoted as almost 95% of children spend approximately 36 weeks in school every year (Simons-Morton, O'Hara, Parcel, Baranowski, & Wilson, 1990). Although quality school physical education programs contribute substantially to children's daily physical activity levels (see Morgan, Beighle, & Pangrazi, 2007), schools have not been able to attenuate the decrease of children's overall physical activity levels. Unfortunately, even if schools mandate over 50% of physical activity class time be spent in moderate-to-vigorous physical activity, accumulating 60 minute of daily moderate-to-vigorous physical activity during these sessions is not possible given the duration of in-class sessions (Corbin, Pangrazi, & Le Masurier, 2004; Morgan, Beighle, & Pangrazi, 2007; National Association for Sport and Physical Education, 2004). Furthermore, among the 80% of schools requiring physical education, only 3.8% of elementary schools, 7.9% of middle schools, and 2.1% of high schools provide daily physical education classes to students (Centers for Disease Control and Prevention, 2005). In response, many children's health advocates call for cooperation from communities and families to promote greater daily physical activity among children (Centers for Disease Control and Prevention, 2000).

Impact of Personal Attributes on Physical Activity

Researchers have reported that children differ in their physical activity levels across different grades and age groups (see Kulinna, Martin, Lai, Kliber, & Reed, 2003; Vincent & Pangrazi, 2002) with children's physical activity levels declining dramatically as they age (U.S. Department of Health and Human Services, 2012). Research has indicated that students' moderate-to-vigorous physical activity increased from nine to 10 years of age, peaked at 11 to 12 years of age, and then decreased in later school years (Vincent & Pangrazi, 2002). The preceding results have been corroborated in other studies as well. Klausen and colleagues indicated physical activity levels in physical education were lower in older children (aged 12 to 13 years) than in younger children (aged 10 to 11 years)(Klausen, Rasmussen, & Schibye, 1986), while Kulinna et al. (2003) found elementary school children displayed the highest physical activity levels, followed by high school and middle school students.

A majority of the findings regarding children's moderate-to-vigorous levels as a function of gender have suggested that boys are more active than girls with only a few studies reporting no differences in physical activity levels between genders (Centers for Disease Control and Prevention, 1996). Research conducted in physical education settings has reported that boys tend to be more active than girls regardless of the type of activity (Vincent & Pangrazi, 2002). For example, research has shown that boys were more active than girls in overall activity levels, skill drills, game play, and free play (Michaud, Cauderay, Narring, & Schutz, 2002). Further, gender differences in physical activity participation appear to manifest themselves in other countries as well. For example, Canadian males aged 10-17 years spent nearly 20% more time in physical activity than did females during out-of-school hours (Castelli & Erwin, 2007). In a study of a wide range of age groups, Asian scholars reported that Taiwanese adolescent girls had lower physical activity levels than boys and that boys were more active than girls in preschool children at ages as young as three years (Wu, Pender, & Noureddine, 2003). Given the fact that girls are generally less physically active than boys, and that physical activity behaviors during adolescence predict obesity during adulthood, the present study was designed to investigate adolescent girls' physical activity participation in the state of New Mexico to address the current status and determinants of physical activity behaviors among this unique, multi-ethnic population.

In comparison to the extensive study of age and gender differences in physical activity which exist within the literature, race/ethnicity differences in physical activity, especially among adolescent girls, have received much less attention. Of the research which has been conducted, findings indicate youth's physical activity levels vary by ethnicity. For instance, studies conducted through the Centers for Disease Control and Prevention of children and adolescents aged 10-17 years indicated that Caucasians' rates of regular physical activity participation were higher than the rates for non-Caucasians (Centers for Disease Control and Prevention, 2006). Specifically, 73.5% and 69.1% of Caucasian and African-American children, respectively, participated in physical activity three and more days per week while only 62.9% Hispanic children engaged in this amount of weekly physical activity (Centers for Disease Control and Prevention, 2006).

Beyond the impact of ethnicity on children's physical activity participation, children's physical activity behaviors may be influenced by the other related factors such as socioeconomic status, parental support, and availability of community physical activity facilities. In another study by the

Centers for Disease Control and Prevention of 10-17 years old youth, it was suggested that youth's participations in three or more days per week of physical activity increased as the family income increased, and that children from families living below the federal poverty level were least likely to participate regularly in physical activity when compared to children above the federal poverty level (Centers for Disease Control and Prevention, 2005). Therefore, there is a need to further explore these underlying factors as they relate to adolescent girls' physical activity participation.

Social Cognitive Determinants of Physical Activity

Regular participation in physical activity may lead to improved psychological and physical well-being. As such, motivating children to participate and adhere to physical activity is very important. To this end, it is critical to understand the specific determinants which may lead children to engage in greater or lesser amounts of physical activity. In physical activity and health, the social cognitive theory has been fruitful in explaining individuals' exercise determinants and behaviors (Bandura, 1986, 1997). The social cognitive theory proposes that behavior, the environment, and the person continuously change and simultaneously influence each other. Therefore, three factors (personal, social, and environmental factors) must be considered when trying to understand individuals' physical activity behaviors.

According to the social cognitive theory, self-efficacy is a major personal factor and refers to beliefs about one's capabilities to learn or perform behaviors at designated levels (Bandura, 1986). In general, individuals who feel efficacious tend to perform well, try new behaviors, and exert effort in those behaviors using challenging and realistic goals. In this accord, self-efficacy has been identified as a key predictor of an individual's physical activity participation (Norman, Schmid, Sallis, Calfas, & Patrick, 2005). For example, in a study by Gao, Xiang, Lee, and Kosma (2011), greater physical activity enjoyment and self-efficacy in a population of adolescents was positively associated with higher physical activity participation. In addition, physical activity-related self-efficacy among adolescents was higher in Caucasian girls when compared to African-Americans girls of similar socioeconomic status and geography (Felton et al., 2002).

Social factors reflect social support from significant others such as parents, peers, and teachers (Norman et al., 2005). Operationally, social support refers to "a wide cross section of concepts including belonging, bonding, and binding; attributes of groups, relationships, and persons; and processes that are social, behavioral, and affective" (Bartlett, Gratton, & Rolf, 2009, p. 1225). In studies with children and youth, social support generally comes from parents and family. In particular, Corbin and Pangrazi (1992) found that parental and family support predicted children's physical activity levels. For example, children of active parents have been found to be approximately six times more active as compared to children of inactive parents (Davison, Cutting, & Birch, 2003). As for environmental factors associated with physical activity, access to safe physical activity environments and social restrictions (e.g., social norms, religious beliefs) are among the most prominent determinants. The operational definition of environment refers to an organism's surrounding conditions, influences, or forces (Katmarzyk & Malina, 1999). Many studies have focused on the relationship between a variety of environmental factors and physical activity behaviors. For instance, physical activity opportunities provided by community-based programs have the potential to increase children's physical activity levels. Katzmarzyk and Malina (1999) identified that participation in community-based sports programs accounted for over 50% of youth's physical activity levels suggesting that more attention needs to be paid to how the influence of other contexts aside from the school physical education environment affect physical activity participation.

Measurement Issues in Physical Activity Levels

Numerous measurement instruments have been used in the assessment of physical activity in populations of adolescent boys and girls. When pedometers were used to monitor number of steps and physical activity duration, boys consistently demonstrated more steps and longer physical activity duration than girls regardless of the type of activity (Bandura, 1986; Michaud et al., 2002). Accelerometer studies reached similar conclusions among children in K-12 physical education classes (Lemura, Andreacci, Carlonas, Klebez, & Chelland, 2000; Trost et al., 2002). Of note is the fact a few studies revealed inconclusive findings when using other forms of physical activity measurement. For example, heart-rate monitors-based studies showed no gender differences in physical activity levels existed between 3rd and 12th graders (Coleman, Saelens, Wiedrich-Smith, Finn, & Epstein, 1997).

Additionally, researchers have reported children's physical activity levels were different between objective instruments and self-reported measurements

(Sallis et al., 1996). For instance, according to Pate et al., (2009), middle school girls' annual physical activity levels decreased 4% when analyzing accelerometer data, but these decreases were 6% to 13% during analysis of self-reported physical activity data. The inconsistencies in the findings may owe to the different objective instruments used to assess physical activity (e.g., sensitivity of specific instrument to capture movement) and the nature of the sample completing a self-report physical activity questionnaire (e.g., memory bias among children). Given that both objective instrumentation and self-report questionnaires are used so frequently within the literature, the closer in agreement these two measurement types, the more valid and reliable the data becomes.

Similar to the national trends, New Mexico children's physical activity levels have decreased over time and are lower than the national average with New Mexico adolescent girls' physical activity and sports participation being among the lowest in the nation (Centers for Disease Control and Prevention, 2005). Further, New Mexico is home to a large Hispanic population comprised of a large number of families with higher poverty levels (U.S. Census Bureau, 2010). Despite the aforementioned facts, no study is available exploring adolescent girls' physical activity participation in this community from a public health perspective.

Therefore, the purpose of this study was to investigate the current status and determinants of physical activity participation in a multi-ethnic sample of adolescent girls' in New Mexico as well as examine the discrepancies between various physical activity measurement techniques in this population. More specifically, this study was guided by three questions: 1) What is the current status of adolescent girls' physical activity participation in New Mexico in relation to national recommendations? 2) Which determinants relate most to adolescent girls' physical levels? and 3) What is the relationship between adolescent girls' pedometer-based and self-reported physical activity levels?

METHODS

Participants

Three-hundred eighty nine participants from five public schools and one pre-college summer program at another school in Albuquerque, New Mexico, voluntarily agreed to participate in this study. Of the original sample, some girls declined to participate in the study, dropped out, or provided invalid data.

This resulted in a final sample size of 217 girls and their parents/guardians (retention rate = 57%).

The final sample included 81 sixth (37.3%), 70 seventh (32.3%), and 66 eighth (30.4%) grade students ranging in age from 10 to 13 years with a mean age of 12 years old. Race/ethnicity characteristics of the sample were as follows: 50.7% Hispanic-American, 29.0% Caucasian, 15.2% African American, 5.1% American Indian and others. The preceding race/ethnicity breakdown was representative of the local population of middle school girls.

Instruments

Three survey questionnaires and one pedometer per girl were administered to measure adolescent girls' physical activity determinants (e.g., age/grade, ethnicity, socioeconomic status, and physical activity-related self-efficacy) and physical activity levels, respectively. Assent and consent forms for participating girls and their parents/ guardians, respectively, were filled out and returned prior to any collection of data.

State and Local Middle School Youth Risk Behavior Survey for Children. The State and Local Middle School Youth Risk Behavior Survey was modified from the 2007 Middle School Youth Risk Behavior Survey (kappa 61%-100%). This survey has acceptable reliability and has been used successfully with study populations of varying demographic characteristics (Centers for Disease Control and Prevention, 2005). For the purposes of this study, the questionnaire was adapted from the 2007 Middle School Youth Risk Behavior Survey and Youth Risk Behavior Surveillance for children. Adolescent girls answered 14 multiple choice questions to discern demographic information and assess the girls' physical activity behaviors. One sample question was "In an average week when you are in school, on how many days do you go to physical education classes?" The responses were *0* to *5* days and scored *1* to *6* with 1 representing 0 days and 6 representing 5 days.

Physical Activity Self-Efficacy. Girls' self-efficacy was measured via two categories adapted from the *Guide for Constructing Self-efficacy Scales* (Cronbach's alpha = 0.92) (Bandura, 2006). The aforementioned two categories items were rated on 100% confidence scales from "0 = *cannot do at all*" to "100 = *highly certain can do.*" The first category, self-efficacy to regulate exercise, had 18 short questions. One sample question was "I am confident in my ability (0 - 100) to perform regular exercise 3 or more times a week when I am feeling anxious." The second category, self-efficacy for leisure time skills and extracurricular activities, had eight short questions, including sports skills, learning dance skills, learning music skills, school newspaper, school government work, school plays, regular physical education activities, and learning team sports. One sample question was "I am confident in my ability (0 - 100) to learn dance skills well." The mean score of all items for each category gave an overall indication of the magnitude of a girl's self-efficacy for participating in a regular exercise routine (category one) and self-efficacy for leisure time skills and extracurricular activities (category two), respectively.

Youth Media Campaign Longitudinal Survey for Parents. Youth Media Campaign Longitudinal Survey for Parents is a telephone-interview survey that was designed by the Centers for Disease Control and Prevention to evaluate the effects of the organization's VERB campaign (Welk et al., 2007). The Youth Media Campaign Longitudinal Survey for Parents demonstrates acceptable intraclass correlation coefficients for the estimation of free-time activity (ICC = 0.60) and total weekly physical activity (ICC = 0.60) (Huhman, Heitzier, & Wong, 2004).

In this study, the Youth Media Campaign Longitudinal Survey was converted to a self-administered survey for participating parents/guardians. The 22 questions in this survey assessed parents/guardians' demographic information (e.g., household income, ethnicity, and number of children), physical activity participation, and attitudes towards their child's physical activity. One sample question was "Now, thinking about the next month, how likely are you to do physical activities with this girl [daughter]?" The four responsive items ranged from extremely likely to not very likely, and were scored *1* to *4* with 1 representing "not very likely" and 4 representing "extremely likely."

Pedometer-based Physical Activity Levels. Adolescent girls' daily physical activity levels in this study were assessed objectively with W4L Neo II pedometers over the course of at least four consecutive school days. Specifically, the W4L Neo II provided data on number of steps and total physical activity duration in minutes. Studies indicate W4L pedometers are valid and reliable in measuring ambulatory physical activity among children and physical activity duration and steps in adolescents (Bassett et al., 2000; Bassett & Strath, 2002).

Procedures

This study was approved by the Human Subject Institutional Review Board at the University of New Mexico. An assent form from each participating girl, a consent form from her parents/guardian, and a signed letter from the parent/guardian in which they granted permission for their daughter to participate were required in the study. The consent forms briefly described the study purpose and the level of participant involvement in addition to providing information regarding data collection anonymity. Although included in the assent and consent forms, information regarding study withdrawal procedures and relevant contacts at the university were included in a separate letter to parents/guardians.

The aforementioned materials were distributed by the principal to the potential participants and their parents/guardians in each participating school at the beginning of the data collection period. After the consent/assent forms were obtained from student participants and their parents/guardians, the principal researcher provided each girl the three study questionnaires and pedometer.

To accurately calibrate the pedometers and address any potential inter-instrumental error, a standardized shake test (i.e., 100 shakes of pedometer to ensure no pedometer was off by more than 5%) was given prior to and after the pedometer data collection. To prevent the accidental reset and loss of pedometer data, all pedometers were sealed with plastic cable ties before being distributed to girls. Each girl wore a sealed W4L Neo II Pedometer from Monday or Tuesday morning through Friday morning attached to the right side of the girls' pants, shorts, belt or waistband (Graser, Pangrazi, & Vincent, 2007). The principal researcher and research assistants arrived at the target schools in the morning before the start of school and met participants in the cafeteria or gym. At this time the researchers downloaded the data to the specific data forms, reset the pedometer to zero, re-sealed each pedometer, and helped the girls put the pedometer in the right position—a process which took less than two minutes.

Data Analyses

To answer the research questions, the following steps were conducted using SPSS 15.0 (SPSS, Inc., Chicago, IL): 1) data from the questionnaires and pedometers were placed into Excel (Microsoft Inc., Redmond, WA) to form a database for export to SPSS; 2) the normality, residual variance of pedometer data, and internal consistency of the self-reported data was confirmed; 3) descriptive analyses of the population's characteristics and physical activity levels from the self-report questionnaires and pedometers were conducted; 4) a series of analysis of variance (ANOVA), multivariate analysis of variance (MANOVA), and multivariate analysis of covariance tests (MANCOVA) with post-hoc multiple comparisons were conducted to identify the relationship between girls' pedometer data (steps per day, minutes per day, and steps per minute) and physical activity determinants (e.g., age, ethnicity, socioeconomic status, and self-efficacy); and 5) Box Plots ware constructed to further surmise the relationship between the self-reported and pedometer-based physical activity levels.

RESULTS

Current Status

Histograms of self-report and pedometer data versus residuals plots indicated the data meet the normality and internal consistency requirements for further analysis. The study participants had mean daily step counts, physical activity duration, and step per minute of 8,137 steps, 75.44 minutes, and 107 steps per minute, respectively. Self-reported weekly moderate physical activity for the sample was 3.97 days with a standard deviation of 2.11 days.

Physical Activity Determinants

Age (ANOVA, $p = 0.47$) and grade (ANOVA, $p = 0.44$) were not found to be significant determinants of daily steps or daily physical activity time in adolescent girls as assessed via pedometers. Conversely, ethnicity was identified as a significant physical activity determinant (ANOVA, $p = 0\ .02$). Specifically, African American girls had greater daily physical activity time than Hispanic and Caucasian girls (see Table 1). However, no significant differences in physical activity time were found between Hispanic and Caucasian girls. Daily mean step counts among different ethnicity groups also demonstrated marginally significant results (ANOVA, $p = 0.047$) (See Table 1). Further, parents' education and household income were not significant determinants in adolescent girls' daily steps (2- way ANOVA, $p =$

0.84 and $p = 0.70$, respectively) or physical activity time (2 way ANOVA, $p = 0.71$ and $p = 0.54$, respectively). Although, of note is the fact that after adjusting for household income and parents' education levels, ethnicity was no longer a significant determinant for girls' daily steps (3-way MANCOVA, $p = 0.162$) and physical activity time (3-way MANCOVA, $p = 0.125$).

Table 1. Pairwise Multiple Comparisons of Steps, Time and Dancing Learning Self-Efficacy to Ethnicity (N = 4)

	Mean			Standard Deviation			p values*		
	Step	Time	Dancing learning self-efficacy	Step	Time	Dancing learning self-efficacy	Step	Time	Dancing learning self-efficacy
White vs. Hispanic	25.955	-2.053	-15.958	419.846	3.737	6.160	1.000	1.000	.063
White vs .AA	-1391.822	15.164*	-24.113*	571.007	5.082	7.776	.094	**.019**	**.014**
White vs. others	-872.690	-5.931	-16.902	868.325	7.728	10.562	1.000	1.000	.670
Hispanic vs. AA**	1417.777*	-13.111*	-8.156	527.410	4.694	7.181	**.047**	**.034**	1.000
Hispanic vs. others	-898.645	-3.877	-.945	840.298	7.479	10.133	1.000	1.000	1.000
AA vs. others	519.131	9.234	7.211	925.138	8.234	11.188	1.000	1.000	37.139

Note: * The mean difference is significant at the .05 level; Adjustment for multiple comparisons: Bonferroni. ** African American.

With regard to physical activity-related self-efficacy, data indicate that girls had moderate self-efficacy for regular physical activity participation (mean = 51.64, standard deviation = 21.56). Precisely, self-efficacy was higher during leisure-time physical activity than regular physical activity: learning sports skills (mean = 76.00, standard deviation = 27.79), learning dancing skills (mean = 73.87, standard deviation = 30.15), and participation in team sports (mean = 89.19, standard deviation = 65.93). Multiple comparisons of adolescent girls' physical activity-related self-efficacy only revealed one significant difference between ethnicities wherein African American girls had significantly higher scores for learning dance skills than Caucasian girls (See Table 1). Regarding the determinants of adolescent girls' physical activity-related self-efficacy, grade level was not found to be a significant predictor

(MANOVA, $p = 0.29$) but age (MANOVA, $p = .06$) and ethnicity (MANOVA, $p = 0.01$) demonstrated marginally significantly and significantly relationships with adolescent girls' physical activity-related self-efficacy, respectively.

Measurement Issues

The fifth question of self-reported survey asked "On how many of the past 7 days did you participate in a physical activity for at least 30 minutes that did not make you sweat or breathe hard, such as fast walking, slow bicycling, skating, pushing a lawn mower, or mopping floors?" This question was meant to assess the adolescent girls' moderate physical activity levels with the item scored on an 8-point Likert scale from *0* to *7* days (1 = 0 days, 8 = 7 days) of physical activity during one week.

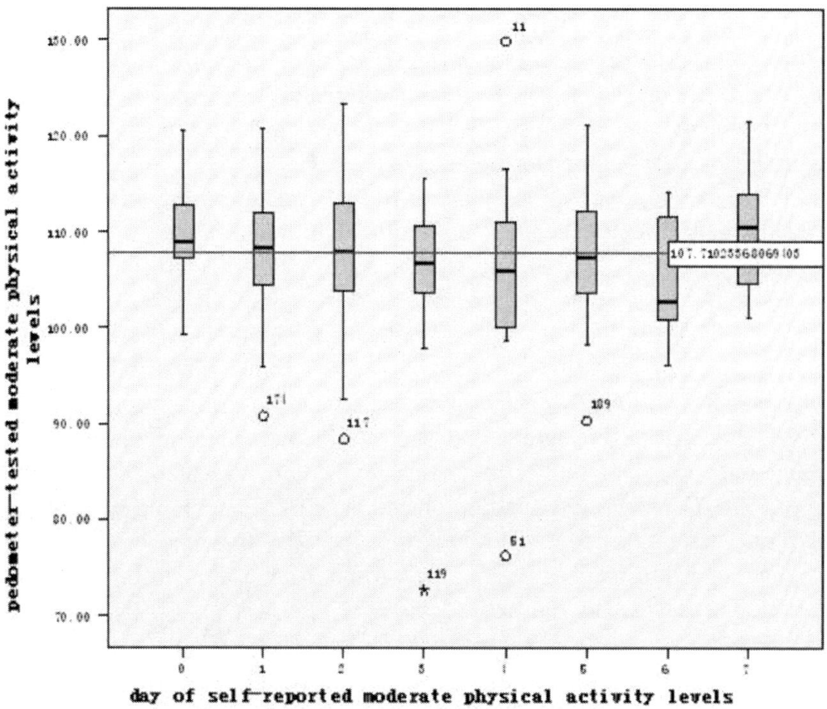

Figure 1. Boxplot of Self-reported and Pedometer-tested Moderate PA (N = 217).

Data on stepper minute suggest that at least 90% of girls in this study reached 107 steps per minute with a narrow range of 98 to 129 steps per minute. This was slightly higher than the 100 steps per minute research has posited as an indicator of moderate physical activity for children (Tudor-Locke et al., 2004). Given this indicator, self-reported days of moderate physical activity and pedometer-assessed moderate physical activity, as assessed by steps per minute equal to or greater than 100, were placed together on a boxplot. As Figure 1 indicates, very little deviation was seen between subjectively and objectively assessed moderate physical activity suggesting a high correlation existed between the subjective and objective measurements of moderate physical activity within the current sample.

Discussion

The purpose of this study was threefold: a) to investigate the current status of adolescent girls' physical activity levels in New Mexico; b) to discern the most significant determinants of adolescent girls' physical activity levels; and c) to examine the relationships between adolescent girls' self-reported physical activity levels and pedometer-based physical activity levels.

With regard to the first research question, the adolescent girls in this study engaged in the recommended duration of physical activity based on pedometer-based data. Specifically, the amount of time adolescent girls spent in daily physical activity participation (75.44 minutes) exceeded the 60 minutes of daily physical activity recommended by the National Association for Sport and Physical Education and the 2008 Physical Activity Guidelines for Americans (National Association for Sports and Physical Education, 2003; Tudor-Locke, Hatano, Pangrazi, & Kang, 2008). Regarding number of steps per day, only 20.3% of study participants reached often recommended 10,000 steps per day (National Association for Sports and Physical Education, 2003). However, literature suggests 10,000 steps per day may not currently be sufficient for youth as obesity continues to be a large and steadily growing concern for today's children and adolescents (Trost et al., 2002). As such, organizations such as the National Association for Sports and Physical Education have recommended youth engage in 11,000 steps per day (See Freedson, Melanson, & Sirard, 1998) meaning only 15.2% of the current sample met these guidelines.

Pertinent to the intensity of adolescent girls' physical activity, the use of pedometers meant no information on physical activity intensity or dose of physical activity was available. Therefore, as has been done in previous studies (Le Masurier, Lee, & Tudor-Locke, 2004; Lioret, Touvier, Lafay, Volatier, & Maire, 2008; Tudor-Locke et al., 2004), 100 steps per minute was stipulated as the minimum standard for moderate physical activity levels. The girls in the present study exceeded this cutoff value, engaging in an average 107 steps per minute (standard deviation = 98 to 129 steps per minute) and, as such, a majority were participating in moderate levels of physical activity. Although, research by Graser et al. (2007) stated that 10-12 year old children should participate in an intensity of physical activity equal to 120-140 steps per minute before physical activity can be classified as moderate to vigorous in intensity. Using Graser et al.'s guidelines for moderate-to-vigorous physical activity, only 4.1% of the current sample met this standard. Although, considering the limitation of pedometers in providing physical activity intensity information, it is warranted that future studies use accelerometry to obtain accurate physical activity intensity data to obtain a more complete view of youth's physical activity patterns (Freedson et al., 1998).

This study also yielded interesting findings regarding adolescent girls' physical activity determinants. To begin, no significant association was seen between adolescent girls' age and grade level and physical activity participation. This finding is somewhat consistent other pedometer-based studies indicating no differences in steps taken between 7th and 8th grade students (Le Masurier et al., 2004) or children of the same gender between the ages of 6 and 12 years (Michaud et al.). However, the present study identified ethnicity to be a significant predictor of adolescent girls' daily physical activity levels. Specifically, African American girls accumulated more steps than Hispanic girls did while also accumulating more daily physical activity time than both Hispanic and Caucasian girls. Yet, the predictive value of ethnicity was no longer significant after controlling for family socioeconomic status and parents' education level.

The finding that adolescent girls' physical activity levels did not differ significantly in regard to ethnicity when controlling for family household income and parents' education levels is noteworthy. Precisely, this finding demonstrates that ethnicity-related differences in adolescent girls' physical activity levels were related more strongly to socioeconomic status variation (which is has a positive association with education levels) than ethnicity. These findings are consistent with studies suggesting a positive association of socioeconomic status on children's physical activity levels (Lioret et al., 2008). Indeed, literature suggests that high socioeconomic status families have the resources to send their daughters to good schools which often have the ability to offer quality school-based physical education and physical activity programs (Gordon-Larsen, Adair, & Popkin, 2002). For example, researchers found that lower physical activity levels in Hispanic and African American adolescent girls were largely attributable to the schools they attended (Richmond, Hayward, Gahagan, Field, & Heisler, 2006). Furthermore, the communities and school districts in which the high socioeconomic status families are located often have more community-based physical activity opportunities (Richmond, Field, & Rich, 2007). Finally, high socioeconomic status families typically have more time available to support and accompany their daughters to participate in physical activities (Biddle, Whitehead, O'Donovan, & Nevill, 2005).

Additionally, while no specific pedometer-based study has been conducted to examine adolescent girls' self-efficacy and daily physical activity levels, researchers have suggested that adolescent girls' physical activity participation is positively associated with self-efficacy. In an attempt to make up for this limitation within the literature, the current study investigated the impact of age, grade, and ethnicity on girls' physical activity-related self-efficacy. Although Felton et al. (2002) indicated that self-efficacy was higher in Caucasian girls than African-American girls when socioeconomic status and geographical factors were similar, our data revealed that girls' general overall physical activity-related self-efficacy did not differ among different ethnicities; however, African American girls reported higher self-efficacy on abilities associated with learning dance than any other ethnicity included in the sample. The authors of the current study speculate that the difference between the present findings and the Felton et al. study arise from: 1) Felton and colleagues controlled for ethnicity which was not done in this study; 2) the use of pedometer-based physical activity measurements in this study and self-reported physical activity measurements in the Felton et al. study; and 3) the wider age range in Felton et al. study. In short, this variation of methodology between studies regarding ethnic differences for physical activity in elementary, middle, and high school girls represents a future research opportunity. This is important as ethnic differences in physical activity mean population-based interventions with the objective of increasing children's physical activity levels will have to determine effective solutions to target different ethnic groups.

Finally, it has been evident that the objective pedometer-tested physical activity levels are different from self-reported results (Kathleen, Lutuchy, Wenthe, & Levy, 2008). According to the flat trend line on Figure 1, we conclude that the self-reported physical activity levels did reflect the actual pedometer data for moderate physical activity (Saris, 1986). This finding is inconsistent with empirical studies in this area of inquiry. Thus, future study should compare more closely the correlation between pedometer and self-report physical activity measurements.

CONCLUSION

Based on the findings from this study, it can be concluded that New Mexico adolescent girls' physical activity participation was strongly associated with family socioeconomic status; although, ethnicity was identified as a related factor of girls' physical activity levels when family socioeconomic status was not taken into account. Indeed, ethnicity is not a factor influencing adolescent girls' physical activity levels, but it is an influential factor predicting some types of self-efficacy (e.g., self-efficacy for learning dance in African American girls). Finally, adolescent girls' self-reported physical activity levels were closely correlated with their pedometer-based physical activity levels. However, more study is needed on comparing pedometer measurements of physical activity to self-reported physical activity measurements among adolescent girls.

The findings of the present study provide substantial evidence indicating the need to further examine the potential factors influencing adolescent girls' physical activity levels, as well as provide practical implications for interventions that will help us promote greater health behaviors among adolescent girls. First, low socioeconomic status girls are at a greater risk of being physically inactive compared to high socioeconomic status girls. Therefore, school educators and health professionals should devote specific efforts to low socioeconomic status populations. Failure to do so could result in a wider socioeconomic status-related health disparity within the education system. Low socioeconomic status girls should be provided more physical activity opportunities, such as extracurricular physical activity opportunities within the schools or communities to help them develop and maintain a healthy lifestyle. Meanwhile, educational resources should be distributed with the health needs of low income school districts in mind. Regardless, more research is needed to explore effective interventions that can promote low socioeconomic status girls' physical activity levels. Finally, enhancing girls' self-efficacy for physical activity within physical education classes might also help increase their physical activity levels in other segments of the day. This is a real challenge for current physical education programs because physical education teachers have been accustomed to teaching only sport movement and skills. As such, physical education teach education programs would benefit from a heavier emphasis on the improvement of psychosocial constructs most relevant to long-term participation in physical activity.

REFERENCES

Ballard, K., Caldwell, D., Dunn, C., Hardison, A., Newkirk, J., Sanderson, M.,…Thomas, C. (2005) *Move More: North Carolina's Recommended Standards For Physical Activity In School*. Raleigh, NC: North Carolina DHHS, Division of Public Health.

Bandura, A. (1986). *Social foundations of thought and action: A social cognitive theory*. Englewood Cliffs, NJ: Prentice Hall.

Bandura, A. (1997). *Self-efficacy: The exercise of control.* New York, NY: WH, Freeman and Company.

Bandura, A. (2006). Guide for constructing self-efficacy scales (pp. 307-337). In Pajares, F, Urdan, T eds. *Self-efficacy beliefs of adolescents*. Greenwich, CT: Information Age Publishing.

Bartlett, R., Gratton, C., & Rolf, C. (2006). *Encyclopedia of international sports studies*. London, England: Routledge.

Bassett, D.R., Ainsworth, B.E., Swartz, A.M., Strath, S.J., O'Brien, W.L., & King, G.A. (2000). Validity of four motions sensors in measuring moderate intensity physical activity. *Medicine and Science in Sport and Exercise, 32*(S9), S471-S480.

Bassett, D.R., & Strath, S.J. (2002). Use of pedometers to assess physical activity (pp. 163-177). In Welk, GJ (eds.). *Physical activity assessments for health-related research.* Champaign, Ill: Human Kinetics.

Biddle S.J.H., Whitehead, S.H., O'Donovan, T.M., & Nevill, M.E. (2005). Correlates of participation in physical activity for adolescent girls: A systematic literature review of recent literature. *Journal of Physical Activity and Health, 2*(4), 423-434.

Castelli, D.M. & Erwin, E.H. (2007). Chapter 4: A comparison of personal attributes and experiences among physically active and inactive children. *Journal of Teaching in Physical Education, 26*, 375-389.

Centers for Disease Control and Prevention. (1996). *U.S. Department of Health and Human Services Physical activity and health: A report of the Surgeon General.* Atlanta, GA: U.S. Department of Health and Human

Services, Centers for Disease Control and Prevention, National Center for Chronic Disease Prevention and Health Promotion.

Centers for Disease Control and Prevention. (2000). Youth risk behavior surveillance-United States, 1999. *Morbidity Mortality Weekly Report, 49*(SS-5), 1–94.

Centers for Disease Control and Prevention. (2005). *The national survey of children's health: Overweight and physical activity among children, a portrait of states and the nation*. Retrieved from: http://mchb.hrsa.gov/overweight/states/newmexico.htm.

Centers for Disease Control and Prevention. (2005). *Youth risk behavior surveillance-United States, 2005 surveillance summaries (Publication No. SS-5)*. Washington, DC: U.S. Government Printing Office.

Coleman, K.J., Saelens, B.E., Wiedrich-Smith, M.D., Finn, J.D., & Epstein, L.H. (1997). Relationships between TriTrac-R3D vectors, heart rate, and self-report in obese children. *Medicine and Science in Sport and Exercise, 29*(11), 1535-1542.

Corbin, C.B. & Pangrazi, P.R. (1992). Are American children and youth fit? *Research Quarterly for Exercise and Sport, 63*(2), 96-106.

Corbin, C.B., Pangrazi, P.R., & Le Masurier, C.G. (2004) Physical activity for children: Current patterns and guidelines. *President's Council on Physical Fitness and Sports Research Digest, 5*(2), 1-8.

Davison, K.K., Cutting, T., & Birch, L. (2003). Parents' activity-related parenting practices predict girls' physical activity. *Medicine and Science in Sport and Exercise, 35*(9), 1589-1595.

Felton, G.M., Dowda, M., Ward, D.S., Dishman, R.K., Trost, S.G., Saunders R., & Pate, R.R. (2002). Differences in physical activity between black and white girls living in rural and urban areas. *Journal of School Health, 72*(6), 250-255.

Freedson, P.S., Melanson, E., & Sirard, J. (1998). Calibration of the Computer Science and Applications, Inc. accelerometer. *Medicine and Science in Sport and Exercise, 30*(5), 777-781.

Gao, Z., Xiang, P., Lee, A.M., & Kosma, M. (2011). Effect of learning activity on students' motivation, physical activity participation and effort/persistence. *International Council for Health, Physical Education, Recreation, Sport, and Dance, 6*(1), 27-33.

Gordon-Larsen, P., Adair, L.S., & Popkin, B.M. (2002). Ethnic differences in physical activity and inactivity patterns and overweight status. *Obesity Research, 10*(3), 141-149.

Graser, S.V., Pangrazi, R.P., & Vincent, J.W. (2007). Effects of placement, attachment, and weight classification on pedometer accuracy. *Journal of Physical Activity and Health, 4,* 359-369.

Hedley, A.A., Ogden, L.C., Johnson, L.C., Carroll, D.M., Curtin, R.L., & Flegal, M.K. (2004). Prevalence of overweight and obesity among U.S. children, adolescents, and adults, 1999-2002. *Journal of the American Medical Association, 291*(23), 2847-2850.

Huhman, M., Heitzier, C., & Wong, F. (2004). The VERB campaign logic model: A tool for planning and evaluation. *Preventing Chronic Disease.* Retrieved from: http://www.cdc.gov/pcd/issues2004/toc.htm.

Kathleen, F.J., Lutuchy, E.M., Wenthe, P., & Levy, M.S. (2008). Measuring activity in children and adolescents using self-report: PAQ-C and PAQ-A. *Medicine and Science in Sport and Exercise, 40*(4), 767-772.

Katmarzyk, P.T., & Malina, R.M. (1999). Contribution of organized sports participation to estimated daily energy expenditure in youth. *Pediatric Exercise Science, 10*, 378-386.

Klausen, K., Rasmussen, B., & Schibye, B. (1986). *Evaluation of the physical activity of school children during a physical education class* (pp. 93-101). In Joseph Rutenfranz, Rolf Mocellin, & Ferdinand Klimt (Eds.). *Children and Exercise XII.* Champaign, IL: Human Kinetics.

Kulinna, P.H., Martin, J., Lai, Q., Kliber, A., & Reed, B. (2003). Student physical activity patterns: Grade, gender and activity influences. *Journal of Teaching in Physical Education, 22*, 298-310.

Le Masurier, G.C., Lee, S.M., & Tudor-Locke, C. (2004). Motion sensor accuracy under controlled and free-living conditions. *Medicine and Science in Sport and Exercise, 36*(5), 905-910.

Lemura, L., Andreacci, J., Carlonas, R., Klebez, J., & Chelland, S. (2000). Evaluation of physical activity measured via accelerometry in rural fourth-grade children. *Perceptual and Motor Skills, 90*, 329-337.

Lioret, S., Touvier, M., Lafay, L., Volatier, J.L., & Maire, B. (2008). Are eating occasions and their energy content related to child overweight and socioeconomic status? *Obesity (Silver Spring), 16*(11), 2518-2523.

Michaud, P.A., Cauderay, M., Narring, F., & Schutz, Y. (2002). Assessment of physical activity with a pedometer and its relationship with VO_2 max among adolescents in Switzerland. *Medicine and Science in Sport and Exercise, 47*(2), 107-115.

Morgan, F.C., Beighle, A., & Pangrazi, R. (2007). What are the contributory and compensatory relationships between physical education and physical activity in children? *Research Quarterly for Exercise and Sport, 78*(5), 407-412.

National Association for Physical Education and Sports. (2003). *Guidelines for appropriate physical activity for elementary school children: Update.* Reston, VA: American Alliance for Physical Activity and Health.

National Association for Sport and Physical Education. (2004). *Physical activity for children: A statement of guidelines for children ages 5-12* (2nd ed.). Reston, VA: American Alliance for Health and Physical Activity.

Norman, G.J., Schmid, B.A., Sallis, J.F., Calfas, K.J., & Patrick, K. (2005). Psychosocial and environmental correlates of adolescent sedentary behaviors. *Pediatrics, 116*, 908-916.

Pate, R.R., Stevens, J., Webber, L.S., Dowda, M., Murray, D.M., Young, D.R., & Going, S. (2009). Age-related change in physical activity in adolescent girls. *Journal of Adolescent Health, 44*(3), 275-282.

Richmond, T.K., Field, A.E., & Rich, M. (2007). Can neighborhoods explain racial/ethnic differences in adolescent inactivity? *International Journal of Pediatric Obesity, 2*(4), 202-210.

Richmond, T.K., Hayward, R.A., Gahagan, S., Field, A.E., & Heisler, M. (2006). Can school income and racial/ethnic composition explain the racial/ethnic disparity in adolescent physical activity participation? *Pediatrics, 117*(6), 2158-2166.

Sallis, J.F., Patrick, K., Harsha; D.W., Feldman, H.A., Ehlinger, S., Stone, E.J.,…Woods, S. (1996). Validation of interviewer- and self- administered physical activity checklists for fifth grade students. *Medicine and Science in Sport and Exercise, 28*(7), 840-851.

Saris, W.H. (1986). Habitual physical activity in children: methodology and findings in health and disease. *Medicine and Science in Sport and Exercise, 18,* 253-263.

Simons-Morton, B.G., O'Hara, G.S., Parcel, T., Baranowski, T., & Wilson, B. (1990). Children's participation in moderate to vigorous physical activity. *Research Quarterly for Exercise and Sport, 61,* 307-314.

Trost, S.G., Pate, R.R., Sallis, J.F., Freedson, P.S., Taylor, W.C., Dowda, M., & Sirard, J. (2002). Age and gender differences in objectively measured physical activity in youth. *Medicine and Science in Sport and Exercise, 34*(2), 350-355.

Tudor-Locke, C., Hatano, Y., Pangrazi, R.P., & Kang, M. (2008). Revisiting "how many steps are enough?." *Medicine and Science in Sport and Exercise, 40*(Suppl. 7), S537-S543.

Tudor-Locke, C., Pangrazi, R.P., Corbin, C.B., Rutherford, W.J., Vincent, S.D., Raustorp, A.,…Cuddihy, T.F. (2004). BMI-referenced standards for recommended pedometer determined steps/day in children. *Preventive Medicine, 38*(6), 857-864.

US Census Bureau. (2010). Federal poverty levels. Retrieved from: http://www.census.gov/hhes/www/poverty/data/incpovhlth/2010/state.xls.

U.S. Department of Health & Human Services. (2012). *Physical Activity Guidelines for Americans Summary*. Retrieved from: http://www.health.gov/paguidelines/guidelines/summary.aspx.

Vincent, D.S. & Pangrazi, P.R. (2002). An examination of the activity patterns of elementary school children. *Pediatric Exercise Science, 14,* 432-41.

Welk, G.J., Wickel, E., Peterson, M., Heitzier, C.D., Fulton, J.E., & Potter, L.D. (2007). Reliability and validity of questions on the youth media campaign longitudinal survey. *Medicine and Science in Sport and Exercise, 39*(4), 612-621.

Wu, T.Y., Pender, N., & Noureddine, S. (2003). Gender differences in the psychosocial and cognitive correlates of physical activity among Taiwanese adolescents: A structural equation modeling approach. *International Journal of Behavioral Medicine, 10*(2), 93-105.

In: Physical Activity Behaviors … ISBN: 978-1-63483-635-7
Editors: Zan Gao and Zachary Pope

Chapter 3

PROTECTION MOTIVATION THEORY-BASED BELIEFS PREDICT ADOLESCENTS' PHYSICAL ACTIVITY AND INTENTION

Charles C. Huang[1,*], Jung Eun Lee[2], Zachary Pope[2] and Zan Gao[2,*]

[1]Wayland Baptist University, Plainview, TX, US
[2]University of Minnesota-Twin Cities, Minneapolis, MN, US

ABSTRACT

According to the protection motivation theory, certain constructs are significantly associated with physical activity intention and behaviors. The purpose of this study was to examine protection motivation theory constructs' predictive strengths on physical activity intention and behavior among adolescents. A total of 222 junior high school students completed a 2-week protection motivation theory-based intervention by reading a leaflet about overweight/obesity and the effects of physical activity on preventing this health threat. Participants' protection motivation theory constructs (response efficacy, response cost, self-efficacy, perceived severity, and perceived vulnerability) and physical activity intention were measured shortly after the intervention. Their self-

* Corresponding Author address: Dr. Zan Gao, 207 Cooke Hall, 1900 University Ave. SE, Minneapolis, MN, 55455 Email: gaoz@umn.edu; Dr. Charles C. Huang, CMB 1227, 1900 West 7th Street, Plainview, TX, 79072 Email: huangc@wbu.edu.

reported physical activity behaviors were measured two weeks later. Hierarchical regression analyses revealed that the entire protection motivation theory model accounted for 14% of variance in adolescents' physical activity behavior. Specifically, intention, perceived vulnerability, and response cost were the significant predictors of adolescents' physical activity behavior. Additionally, protection motivation theory constructs explained 40% of variance in physical activity intention. Self-efficacy and response cost emerged as significant predictors of physical activity intention. The findings provide evidence for the effectiveness of using protection motivation theory as a framework for physical activity intervention implementation among adolescents. Physical activity interventions should concentrate on providing positive coping information to improve adolescents' physical activity self-efficacy and their beliefs about physical activity benefits, as well as minimizing their perception of physical activity cost.

Keywords: response efficacy, response cost, self-efficacy, perceived severity, perceived vulnerability

INTRODUCTION

It has been well-documented that regular participation in physical activity (PA) has a positive influence on individuals' health and well-being (Roberts & Barnard, 2005). Children and adolescents who are more physically active have lower risk of chronic diseases such as obesity and type 2 diabetes (Strong et al., 2005). It has been recommended that adolescents engage in moderate-to-vigorous physical activity for at least 60 minutes daily for enhanced health benefits and weight control (Biddle, Gorely, & Stensel, 2004; Cavill, Biddle, & Sallis, 2001; Strong et al., 2005). However, reports indicate that 92% of adolescents are not meeting the recommended 60 minutes daily physical activity guideline (Troiano et al., 2008). Further, physical activity levels decline as children age, and a substantial number of adolescents are not sufficiently active (Biddle, et al., 2004; Sallis, 2000). Thus, it would be of considerable value to design interventions that promote higher physical activity levels among youth.

The revised protection motivation theory (Rogers, 1983) has the potential to account for the cognitive processes that mediate the behavioral outcomes and the major determinants of physical activity participation, particularly in the context of health-protective behaviors. Many studies have suggested the protection motivation theory to be useful in the prediction of health-related behaviors during interventions (Floyd, Prentice-Dunn, & Rogers, 2000; Milne, Sheeran, & Orvell, 2000; Plotnikoff & Trinh, 2010; Rogers, 1975, 1983).

The protection motivation theory was originally developed in 1975 by Ronald Rogers in an attempt to explain the mechanisms behind individuals' attitudinal and behavioral change when faced with a real or perceived threat to their health (Rogers, 1975). The most recent full model is described in Figures 1 and 2 (Rogers, 1983; Rogers et al., 1997). Rogers (1983) proposed that various environmental (e.g., fear appeals) and intrapersonal (e.g., personality) sources of information is obtained before cognitive mechanisms are initiated. A cognitive mediating process begins once information about a health threat is received. Then, individuals will engage in one of two types of responses based off of cognitive evaluation: a maladaptive response and an adaptive response. When engaging in the maladaptive response, one employs a threat appraisal process, which results from an individual judging the intrinsic and extrinsic rewards associated with the unhealthy alternative (e.g., playing video games rather than completing planned exercise) as being lower than his/her perceptions of the severity of the threat and perceived vulnerability to the threat. The theory inferred that as perceived vulnerability and severity increase, the likelihood of engaging in the unhealthy alternative decreases. However, the likelihood of continuing the unhealthy behavior increases as the perceived intrinsic rewards (e.g., enjoyment, pleasure) and extrinsic rewards for that behavior (e.g., approval by peers; Rogers, 1983) is increased.

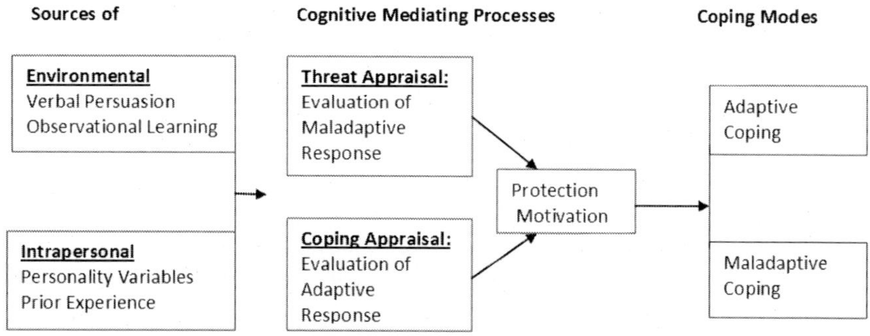

Adapted from Rogers et al., 1997.

Figure 1. Overall Model of Protection Motivation Theory.

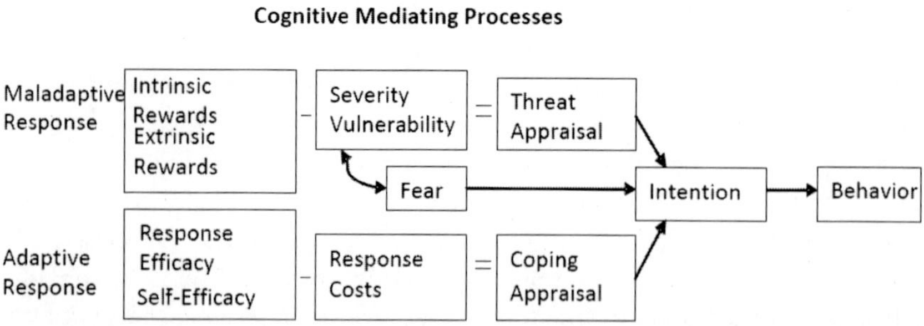

Adapted from Rogers, 1983; Rogers et al., 1997.

Figure 2. Cognitive Mediating Processes of Protection Motivation Theory.

One employing an adaptive response will engage in a coping appraisal. The coping appraisal process is a cognitive process whereby an individual values a coping strategy and the ability to avert the dangers of a given threat. This form of appraisal results from an individual's favorable perception of response efficacy (i.e., physical activity will lead to weight lost in addition to decreasing the risk of obesity-related diseases effectively) and self-efficacy (i.e., the belief in one's personal ability to complete physical activity) when considering the perceived costs of completing the adaptive response (i.e., physical activity). Response efficacy is the perception that a particular coping strategy will effectively work to avoid the dangers of the threat. Self-efficacy refers to one's own belief regarding his/her capability to effectively carry out the adaptive response. Response cost, on the other hand, inhibits performance of the adaptive behavior. Response cost can be any cost (e.g., physical, psychological, social, monetary) that might reduce the probability of using the adaptive response. According to protection motivation theory, people's intention to adopt an adaptive response (protection motivation) is the function of an individual's threat appraisal and coping appraisal. However, most research and applications of the protection motivation theory examine the effects of five main constructs (perceived severity, perceived vulnerability, self-efficacy, response efficacy, and response cost) (Lippke & Plotnikoff, 2009; Milne, Orbell, & Sheeran, 2002; Plotnikoff & Trinh, 2010; Zhang & Cooke, 2011).

Two meta-analyses (Floyd et al., 2000; Milne et al., 2000) and two reviews (Norman, Boer, & Seydel, 2005; Plotnikoff et al., 2010) have summarized the findings from studies that examined protection motivation theory across various behaviors, with most studies indicating the protection motivation theory to be moderately effective in predicting health-related and safety-related intentions and behaviors. Specifically, studies have shown modest support for both threat appraisal and coping appraisal constructs of the this theory in predicting health-related intentions and behaviors, with coping appraisal constructs emerging as the strongest predictors (Floyd et al., 2000; Milne et al., 2000; Norman, Boer, & Seydel, 2005; Plotnikoff & Trinh, 2010). For example, Sturges and Rogers (1996) examined how youth and adults reacted to the health threats caused by smoking and their ability to cope by abstaining from smoking. They concluded that the greatest change in intention occurred when self-efficacy and response efficacy to abstain from smoking were high in a situation where health threat and severity were also high.

Protection motivation theory has also been employed in the physical activity domain. Plotnikoff and Higginbotham (2002) found that the coping appraisal constructs had strong positive associations with exercise intention while the threat appraisal (for heart disease) constructs had limited association with the exercise outcomes. Specifically, fear was weakly associated with intention, whereas vulnerability was negatively associated with intentions and behavior. In another study by the same researchers, Plotnikoff and Higginbotham (1998) indicated that self-efficacy was strongly associated with low-fat diet intentions and exercise intentions. Plotnikoff et al., (2009) also examined the utility of protection motivation theory to predict physical activity behavior in a longitudinal study over two consecutive 6-month periods. The results showed that both self-efficacy and response efficacy were significantly associated with intention and behavior, while self-efficacy and intentions significantly predicted subsequent physical activity behavior.

Some research was interested in examining this theory in the primary care setting as well. Tulloch and colleagues (2009) examined the utility of protection motivation theory in the prediction of exercise intentions and behavior among cardiac patients and found that most of the protection motivation theory constructs (perceived severity, response efficacy, and self-efficacy) predicted exercise intentions, which, in turn predicted exercise behavior. However, the protection motivation theory model was not reliable for predicting exercise behaviors at 12 months after hospitalization. Similarly, Blanchard and associates (2009) tested protection motivation theory in explaining exercise intentions and behavior in cardiac patients receiving a home-based cardiac rehabilitation program. They concluded that threat appraisal constructs had limited motivational influence on exercise levels in home-based cardiac rehabilitation patients, whereas coping appraisal constructs were useful in explaining exercise behavior in this population. Finally, a study by Plotnikoff et al., (2010) examined protection motivation theory in the context of diabetes management, and revealed that coping appraisal constructs significantly predicted intention and behavior in both type 1 and type 2 diabetes groups, with self-efficacy being the strongest predictor. Among threat appraisal constructs, only severity significantly contributed to the explanation of the variance in intention in the type 2 diabetes group; and vulnerability was not significantly related to physical activity intention or behavior. Among coping appraisal constructs, self-efficacy and intention were significantly associated with physical activity behavior.

Seven studies explored the effects of manipulating specific constructs regarding the cognitive process related to protection motivation theory constructs, intention, and behavior (Courneya & Hellsten, 2001; Fruin et al., 1991; Graham, Prapavessis, & Cameron, 2006; Milne et al., 2002; Stanley & Maddux, 1986; Wurtele & Maddux, 1987; Zhang et al., 2011). All studies implemented interventions to manipulate the theory constructs using motivational essays or videos. These interventions primarily emphasized the prevention of health risks through physical activity or exercise. The findings of these studies indicated that the interventions were generally effective in influencing subsequent cognitions and intention. However, as Milne et al., (2000) illustrated in a review, the effectiveness of these interventions in influencing subsequent behavior was limited.

Among the aforementioned seven studies, three studies (Graham et al., 2006; Milne et al., 2002; Zhang et al., 2011) employed a factual health education intervention to examine the usefulness of the protection motivation theory on behavioral intentions revealing mixed findings. Specifically, in a study by Graham et al., 2006, the intervention group received information regarding the susceptibility and severity of colon cancer, evidence linking colon cancer and exercise, and some common methods to help increase one's response efficacy and self-efficacy for engaging in more exercise. The intervention group's early exercise behavior was improved (two weeks post-intervention) but their longer term exercise behavior (four weeks post-intervention) did not show any improvement. In another study (Milne et al., 2002), the intervention group was asked to read a health education leaflet based on protection motivation theory constructs, containing factual information about coronary heart disease and the benefits of exercise. This intervention group significantly increased threat and coping appraisal and intentions to engage in exercise but did not reveal a significant increase in subsequent exercise behavior. Zhang et al., (2011) also reported in a similar study that a protection motivation theory-based intervention had significant positive effects on protection motivation theory constructs, intentions, and the physical activity behavior. Thus, further research is warranted to seek the best ways of intervening with factual health education interventions to promote more favorable cognitive processes related to protection motivation theory constructs as well as physical activity intention and behavior.

The purposes of this study were to examine the predictive strengths of protection motivation theory constructs on physical activity intention and behavior among adolescents, and to determine whether weight status moderates the relationships between protection motivation theory constructs and physical activity intention and behavior. It was hypothesized that protection motivation theory constructs will significantly predict adolescents' physical activity intention and physical activity behavior.

METHODS

Participants

The participating school was a suburban public school in the Mountain West Region of the United States. There were 412 seventh through ninth grade students enrolled in 12 physical education classes with class size ranging from 28 to 40 students. In the present study, 226 students agreed to participate. The age of the sample ranged 12 -15 years old, and the mean age was 13.4 years old (SD = 0.95). The sample consisted of 34.7% seventh grade, 37.4% eighth grade, and 27.9% ninth grade students. Ethnic backgrounds of the participants were 75.2% White American, 7.7% Hispanic American, 3.6% African American, 1.8% Asian American, and 11.7% others.

Two experienced physical education teachers (one male and one female) taught the physical education classes. Seventh grade students had been introduced to a variety of sports. The emphasis in the physical education class was being physically active and having fun. Eighth and ninth grade students continued to practice sports-related skills. Physical education classes focused on accruing physical activity, learning individual and team sport strategies and fostering teamwork.

Permission to conduct the study was obtained from the University Institutional Review Board, the district, the school administration, and the physical education teachers prior to the implementation of this study. Students and parents provided written informed assent and consent form, respectively, prior to participation in this study. Finally, this study involved the measures of protection motivation theory constructs shortly after the intervention (Time 1) and the measures of participants' self-reported physical activity behavior two weeks later (Time 2).

Instruments

Demographics. Students self-reported gender, age, grade, and race. The students' height was measured by a Seca Stadiometer (Accurate to .1 cm, Seca Corp, CA) and weight was measured by a Taylor Digital Scale (Accurate to .1 kg, Model 7340B, Taylor Precision Products, Oak Brook, IL).

Motivational intervention materials. Two separate leaflets were produced for this study. The first leaflet was designed to incorporate the five major constructs of protection motivation theory: perceived severity, perceived vulnerability, response efficacy, self-efficacy, and response cost. The leaflet contained factual information about the prevalence and nature of overweight/obesity and the effects of physical activity on preventing this health threat. The content validity of this leaflet was confirmed by five health education specialists (two professors and three school health education teachers). All specialists agreed that the leaflet contained major relevant information and made minor revisions to the leaflet. All the protection motivation theory constructs were modified from the Milne et al., (2002) version based on the condition of interest in this study (overweight/obesity as the health threat as opposed to coronary heart disease). Participants in both of the two experimental groups were told that: "The following passage presents a true account of the effect of physical activity on reducing the risk of overweight/obesity." The leaflet expanded on the following protection motivation theory constructs:

1) *Perceived severity* consisted of statements outlining the physical, psychological, and social consequences of overweight/obesity.
2) *Perceived vulnerability* consisted of statements describing that adolescents who do not participate in physical activity are very likely to develop overweight/obesity in the future.
3) *Response efficacy* consisted of statements explaining the effectiveness of physical activity in preventing overweight/obesity.
4) *Self-Efficacy* consisted of statements suggesting that it would be easy for participants to engage in physical activity.
5) *Response cost* consisted of the statement: "Although adopting regular physical activity does have its costs, most adolescents find these to be

> very minor and easily overcome and find that the benefits of regular physical activity far outweigh the costs."

A second leaflet was produced for the attention control condition. It was the opening paragraphs of a novel and was in similar length to the first leaflet but had content unrelated to physical activity (King, 2011).

Protection motivation theory constructs and intention. The constructs and intention measures were assessed on 5-point Likert scales, comprising belief statements coupled with appropriate response items. All the items were randomized so that patterns of questions were less obvious to the students (Sheeran & Orbell, 1996). Perceived severity was measured by one item, namely, 'If I were to develop overweight/obesity I would suffer a lot of health problems (*strongly disagree—strongly agree*).' Perceived vulnerability was measured by two items, such as, 'My chances of developing overweight/obesity in the future are (*not at all strong—very strong*).' Response efficacy was measured by one item, namely, 'Participating in physical activity at least 60 minutes daily is a good way of reducing the risk of developing overweight/obesity (*strongly disagree—strongly agree*).' Self-efficacy was measured by four items, such as, 'I feel confident in my ability to participate in physical activity at least 60 minutes daily in the next two weeks (*strongly agree—strongly disagree*).' Response cost was measured by four items, such as, 'The benefits of taking physical activity for 60 minutes daily outweigh the costs (*strongly agree—strongly disagree*).' Physical activity intention was measured by two items, such as, 'I do not wish to participate in physical activity at least 60 minutes daily in the next two weeks (*strongly agree—strongly disagree*).' To score each construct, the scores for items that were reverse scored were first recoded. Then, the mean score for all items for each construct were calculated. All the protection motivation theory constructs and intention that were measured by multiple items formed reliable scales, with Cronbach's α values ranging from .73 to .95 (Milne et al., 2002).

Physical activity levels. Self-reported physical activity behavior has been shown previously to be reliable and correlated with accelerometer data in adolescents (Prochaska, Sallis, & Long, 2001). A two-item overall physical activity questionnaire (Durant et al., 2008) was employed in this study. Students were asked, 'How many days in a typical week were you physically active for at least 60 minutes?' and 'How many days in the past week were you physically active for at least 60 minutes?' These two items were averaged to obtain a measure of moderate to vigorous physical activity. Moderate reliability (intraclass correlation = .61) has been demonstrated in adolescents aged 12-18 years who attended schools outside of their home (Durant et al., 2008).

Body weight category. Participants' body weight and height were measured to calculate their body mass index and determine body weight category. Body mass index is a measure used to determine childhood overweight and obesity in large scale studies. The Centers for Disease Control and Prevention Growth Charts (Centers for Disease Control and Prevention, 2011) were used to determine the corresponding body mass index-for-age and sex percentile. For children and adolescents (aged 2-19 years), overweight is defined as a body mass index at or above the 85th percentile and lower than the 95th percentile; Obesity is defined as a body mass index at or above the 95th percentile for children or adolescents of the same age and sex. Table 1 lists the Centers for Disease Control and Prevention cut-off points for body mass index for overweight and obesity by gender between 11 and 15 years.

Table 1. CDC BMI Cut-off Points for Overweight/Obesity by Gender between 11 and 15 Years

	Underweight		Overweight		Obesity	
Age	Boys	Girls	Boys	Girls	Boys	Girls
11	14.5	14.3	20.2	20.8	23.2	24.2
12	15.0	14.8	21.0	21.7	24.2	25.2
13	15.4	15.3	21.8	22.5	25.2	26.2
14	16.0	15.8	22.6	23.3	26.0	27.2
15	16.5	16.3	23.4	24.0	26.8	28.1

Data Analyses

A correlation matrix was produced in order to determine zero-order relationships between each protection motivation theory construct, physical activity intention, and physical activity behavior. The strength and direction of a linear relationship between any two aforementioned variables without controlling any other variables would be confirmed. To test protection motivation theory constructs' predictive ability on physical activity intention and physical activity behavior, two hierarchical regression analyses with forced entry were employed. Time 1 cognitive processes related to protection motivation theory constructs and physical activity intention were measured immediately after the intervention and self-reported physical activity behavior at Time 2 was measured two weeks after the intervention. Thus, Time 1 cognitive processes related to protection motivation theory constructs and physical activity intention were used to predict Time 2 physical activity behavior; and Time 1 cognitive process related to protection motivation theory constructs were used to predict Time 1 physical activity intention. To determine the association of the protection motivation theory constructs and physical activity intention with physical activity behavior in the first analysis, intention was regressed onto physical activity behavior in Block 1; and then self-efficacy, response efficacy, response cost, perceived severity, and perceived vulnerability were regressed onto behavior in Block 2. In order to determine whether the weight category moderated the relationships between protection motivation theory constructs and physical activity behavior, weight category × self-efficacy, weight category × response efficacy, weight category × response cost, weight category × perceived severity, and weight category × vulnerability were entered in Block 3. Next, the second hierarchical regression analysis was used to determine the association of the protection motivation theory constructs with physical activity intentions. Self-efficacy, response efficacy, response cost, perceived severity, and perceived vulnerability were entered in Block 1. Weight category × self-efficacy, weight category × response efficacy, weight category × response cost, weight category × perceived severity, and weight category × perceived vulnerability were entered in Block 2.

RESULTS

Two hundred twenty two students completed the study. Descriptive statistics and correlations among each of the variables are presented in Table 2. Intention ($r = 0.23$, $p < 0.01$), self-efficacy ($r = .24$, $p < 0.01$), response efficacy ($r = .18$, $p < 0.01$), response cost ($r = - 0.28$, $p < 0.01$), and perceived vulnerability ($r = - 0.23$, $p < 0.01$) were significantly correlated with physical activity behavior. Additionally, self-efficacy ($r = 0.52$, $p < 0.01$), response efficacy ($r = 0.20$, $p < 0.01$), response cost ($r = - 0.57$, $p < 0.01$), and perceived vulnerability ($r = - 0.14$, $p < 0.05$) were significantly correlated with physical activity intention.

Table 2. Descriptive Statistics and Correlations among Variables

	2	3	4	5	6	7	*Mean*	*SD*
1. Physical activity	.23**	.24**	.18**	-.28**	-.05	-.23**	4.80	1.37
2. Intention		.52**	.20**	-.57**	.06	-.14*	4.07	1.01
3. Self-Efficacy			.18**	-.51**	.09	-.24**	3.85	.84
4. Response Efficacy				-.20**	.13*	-.09	4.66	.60
5. Response Cost					-.13*	.13*	1.91	.77
6. Perceived Severity						.06	4.43	.76
7. Vulnerability							2.19	.99

Notes. $*p < .05$; $**p < .01$

Table 3. Models Predicting Physical Activity Behavior

	F_{change}	R^2	R^2_{change}	B^1	B^2	B^3	β^1	β^2	β^3
(Block 1)	12.45**	.06	.06						
Intention				.32**	.08	.05	.23**	.06	.03
(Block 2)	4.20**	.14	.08						
Self-Efficacy					.11	-.01		.07	-.00
Response Efficacy					.26	-.26		.11	-.11
Response Cost					-.31*	-.34*		-.18*	-.20*
Perceived Severity					-.15	.04		-.08	-02
Perceived Vulnerability					-.22*	-.30*		-.16*	-.22*
(Block 3)	1.81	.17	.03						
Weight × Self-Efficacy						.54			.72
Weight × Response Efficacy						-.10			.15
Weight × Response Cost						.09			.07
Weight × Perceived Severity						-.55			-.84
Weight × Perceived Vulnerability						-.20			.20

Notes. B^{1-3} and β^{1-3}= unstandardized and standardized regression coefficients for model 1-3.$*p < .05$; $**p < .01$

Table 4. Models Predicting Physical Activity Intention

	F_{change}	R^2	R^2_{change}	B^1	B^2	β^1	β^2
(Block 1)	28.35**	.40	.40				
Self-Efficacy				.37**	.31**	.30**	.25**
Response Efficacy				.11	.29*	.07	.17*
Response Cost				-.52**	-.56**	-.40**	-.43**
Perceived Severity				-.04	-.05	-.03	-.03
Perceived Vulnerability				-.00	-.05	-.00	-.05
(Block 2)	1.96	.42	.02				
Weight × Self-Efficacy					.28		.51
Weight × Response Efficacy					-.42		-.90
Weight × Response Cost					.14		.14
Weight × Perceived Severity					.01		.02
Weight × Perceived Vulnerability					.17		.24

Notes. B^{1-2} and β^{1-2}= unstandardized and standardized regression coefficients for model 1and model 2.
*$p < .05$; **$p < .01$

To predict physical activity behavior, the results of the hierarchical regression analysis revealed that the entire protection motivation theory constructs accounted for 14% of variance, with intention accounting for 6% (F (1, 220) = 12.45, $R^2 = 0.06$, $p < 0.01$ for model 1 of predicting behavior) and protection motivation theory constructs accounting for 8% (F (5, 215) = 4.20, $R^2 = 0.14$, $p < 0.01$ for model 2 of predicting behavior; Table 3). Specifically, in Block 1, intention was a significant predictor of physical activity behavior ($\beta = 0.23$ $p < 0.01$). In Block 2, the protection motivation theory constructs of response cost ($\beta = -0.18$, $p < 0.05$) and perceived vulnerability ($\beta = -0.16$, $p < 0.05$) were the significant predictors of physical activity behavior. The weight category as moderator in Block 3 was not statistically significant (F (5,210) = 1.81, $R^2_{change} = 0.03$, $p > 0.05$).

In terms of physical activity intention, regression analysis revealed that the protection motivation theory constructs (F (5, 216) = 28.35, $R^2 = 0.40$, $p < 0.01$ for model 1 for predicting intention) accounted for 40% of the variance in physical activity intention (see Table 4). Specifically in Block 1, self-efficacy ($\beta = 0.30$, $p < 0.01$) and response cost ($\beta = -0.40$, $p < 0.01$) were significant predictors of physical activity intention. Weight category was the moderator in the relationship between protection motivation theory constructs and physical activity intention in Block 2 was not statistically significant (F (5,211) = 1.96, $R^2_{change} = 0.03$, $p > 0.05$).

DISCUSSION

The purpose of this study was to test the protection motivation theory in predicting physical activity intention and physical activity behavior among adolescents, and to determine whether weight category moderates relationships between protection motivation theory constructs and physical activity intention or physical activity behavior.

This study found that physical activity intention and response cost were significant predictors of physical activity behavior, and that self-efficacy and response cost were significant predictors of physical activity intention. The findings are partially in line with the results of previous studies which concluded that coping appraisal constructs (self-efficacy, response efficacy, response cost) were significantly associated with physical activity intention and behavior (Fruin et al., 1991; Plotnikoff & Higginbotham, 2002; Plotnikoff et al., 2009; Tulloch et al., 2009; Wurtele et al., 1987). A meta-analysis (Floyd et al., 2000) revealed that coping appraisal constructs (especially self-efficacy) were the strongest predictors of protection motivation (i.e., intention) and behavior. However, in this study self-efficacy was not a significant predictor associated with physical activity behavior. It could be due to the possibility that students already had high self-efficacy and this ceiling effect attenuated the strength of the relationship. Among the other findings, the negative association between response cost and physical activity intention and physical activity behavior, is consistent with other previous studies. For example, Floyd et al., (2000) conducted a meta-analysis of 65 studies and reported a medium effect size for response cost. Referring to statements of response cost items in the protection motivation theory questionnaire, this finding implies that adolescents did not feel physical activities interfered with their spare time or that too many other activities are perceived as more excited and desired.

The finding of a significant association between physical activity intentions and behavior is consistent with previous studies. Researchers have asserted that behavioral intentions predict actual behaviors (Ajzen & Fishbein, 1980; Plotnikoff et al., 2002). In addition, a meta-analysis (Milne et al., 2000) revealed that the largest association in the protection motivation theory framework is demonstrated between intention and behavior. Intention appears to have an average of medium-to-strong correlation with subsequent behavior. Thus, it can be inferred that intention is the best and most immediate predictor of behavior in the protection motivation theory model.

The results of the current study also showed that perceived vulnerability was negatively associated with physical activity behavior. The findings are partially consistent with previous studies in the field of physical activity. Although protection motivation theory proposed that perceived vulnerability should be positively related to health-protective intentions and behavior, studies on physical activity demonstrated limited or inconsistent associations between perceived vulnerability and physical activity behavior (Norman et al., 2005; Plotnikoff & Higginbotham, 2002; Wurtle & Maddux, 1987). In fact, in some studies, negative correlations between perceived vulnerability and health-related behaviors were found (Ben-Ahron et al., 1995; Plotnikoff & Higginbottom, 1998; Seydel et al., 1990). This negative association might be explained by "defensive avoidance" coping styles (Rogers, 1983; Seydel et al., 1990). In other words, when individuals feel vulnerable to a health threat, they become more anxious and thereby engage in various maladaptive coping responses to deal with the anxiety associated with threat (e.g., denial, avoidance). Another possible explanation for the negative association between perceived vulnerability and physical activity behavior is that individuals could have already taken precautions (e.g., physical activity) to avoid a certain health threat, of which decreases perceived vulnerability to the threat. Based on the low score of perceived vulnerability in the present study, the negative association of perceived vulnerability with physical activity behavior might be due to the latter explanation, students having taken precautions.

In conclusion, there was a significant association between adolescents' physical activity behavior and response cost, perceived vulnerability and physical activity intention. Adolescents' physical activity intention was also significantly predicted by self-efficacy and response cost.

REFERENCES

Ajzen, I. & Fishbein, M. (1980). *Understanding attitudes and predicting social behavior*. Englewood Cliffs, NJ: Prentice-Hall.

Ben-Ahron, V., White, D., & Phillips, K. (1995). Encouraging drinking at safe limits on single occasions: the potential contribution of protection motivation theory, *Alcohol and Alcoholism, 30*, 633-639.

Biddle, S. J. H., Gorely, T., & Stensel. (2004). Health-enhancing physical activity and sedentary behavior in children and adolescents. *Journal of Sports Sciences, 22*, 679-701.

Cavill, N., Biddle, S., & Sallis, J. F. (2001). Health enhancing physical activity for young people: Statement of the United Kingdom Expert Consensus Conference. *Pediatric Exercise Science, 13*, 12-25.

Centers for Disease Control and Prevention. (2011). *About BMI for children and teens.,* Retrieved from http://www.cdc.gov/healthyweight/assessing/bmi/childrens_bmi/about_childrens_bmi.html.

Courneya, K.S., & Hellsten, L.A.M. (2001). Cancer prevention as a source of exercise motivation: An experimental test using protection motivation theory. *Psychology, Health and Medicine, 6*(1), 59-64.

Durant, N., Harris, S.K., Doyle, S., Person, S., Saelens, B.E., Kerr, J., … Sallis, J.F. (2008). Relation of school environment and policy to adolescent physical activity. *Journal of School Health, 79*, 153-159.

Floyd, D.L., Prentice-Dunn, S., & Rogers, R.W. (2000). A meta-analysis of research on protection motivation theory. *Journal of Applied Social Psychology, 30*(2), 407-429.

Fruin, D.J., Pratt, C., & Owen, N. (1991). Protection motivation theory and adolescents' perceptions of exercise. *Journal of Applied Social Psychology, 22*(1), 55-69.

Graham, S.P., Prapavessis, H., & Cameron, L.D. (2006). Colon cancer information as a source of exercise motivation. *Psychology and Health, 21*(6), 739-755.

King, A.S. (2011). *Everybody sees the ants*. New York: Little and Brown Company.

Lippke, S., & Plotnikoff, R.C. (2009). The protection motivation theory within the stages of the transtheoretical model – State-specific interplay of variables and prediction of exercise stage transitions. *British Journal of Health Psychology, 14*, 211-229.

Milne, S., Orbell, S., & Sheeran, P. (2002). Combining motivational and volitional interventions to promote exercise participation: Protection motivation theory and implementation intentions. *British Journal of Health Psychology, 7*, 163-184.

Milne, S., Sheeran, P., & Orbell, S. (2000). Prediction and intervention in health-related behavior: A meta-analytic review of protection motivation theory. *Journal of Applied Social Psychology, 30*(1), 106-143.

Norman, P., Boer, H., & Seydel, E. (2005). Protection motivation theory. In M. Conner, & P. Norman (Eds.), *Predicting health behavior: Research and practice with social cognition models* (2nd ed.; pp 81-126). London: Open University Press.

Plotnikoff, R.C., & Higginbotham, N. (1998). Protection motivation theory and the prediction of exercise and low-fat diet behaviors among Australian cardiac patients. *Psychology and Health, 13*, 411-429.

Plotnikoff, R.C., & Higginbotham, N. (2002). Protection motivation theory and exercise behavior change for the prevention of heart disease in a high-risk, Australian representative community sample of adults. *Psychology, Health and Medicine, 7*(1), 87-98.

Plotnikoff, R.C., Lippke, S., Trinh, L., Courneya, K., Birkett, N., & Sigal, R. (2010). Protection motivation theory and the prediction of physical activity among adult with type 1 or type 2 diabetes in a large population sample. *British Journal of Health Psychology, 15,* 643-661.

Plotnikoff, R.C., Rhodes, R.E., & Trinh, L. (2009). Protection motivation theory: A longitudinal test among a representative population sample of Canadian adults. *Journal of Health Psychology, 14* (8), 1119-1134.

Plotnikoff, R.C., & Trinh, L. (2010). Protection motivation theory: Is this a worthwhile theory for physical activity promotion? *Exercise and Sport Sciences Reviews, 38*(2), 91-98.

Plotnikoff, R.C., Trinh, L., Courneya, K.S., Kanunamuni, N., & Sigal, R.J. (2009). Predictors of aerobic physical activity and resistance training among Canadian adults with type 2 diabetes: An application of the protection motivation theory. *Psychology of Sport and Exercise, 10*(3), 320-328.

Prochaska, J.J., Sallis, J.F., & Long, B. (2001). A physical activity screening measure for use with adolescents in primary care. *Archives of Pediatrics & Adolescent Medicine, 155*(5), 554-559.

Roberts, C.K., & Barnard, R.J. (2005). Effect of exercise and diet on chronic disease. *Journal of Applied Physiology, 98(1)*, 3-30.

Rogers, R.W. (1975). A protection motivation theory of fear appeals and attitude change. *Journal of Psychology, 91*(1), 93-114.

Rogers, R.W., & Prentice-Dunn, S. (1997). Protection motivation theory. In D. Gochman (Ed.), *Handbook of health behavior research 1: Personal and social determinants* (pp. 113-132). New York: Plenum.

Rogers, R.W. (1983). Cognitive and physiological processes in fear-based attitude change: A revised theory of protection motivation. In J. Cacioppo & R. Petty (Eds.), *Social psychophysiology: A sourcebook* (pp. 153-176). New York, NY: Guilford.

Sallis, J. F. (2000). Age-related decline in physical activity: A synthesis of human and animal studies. *Medicine and Science in Sports and Exercise, 23*, 1598-1600.

Seydel, E., Taal, E., & Wiegman, O. (1990). Risk-appraisal, outcome and self-efficacy expectancies: Cognitive factors in preventive behavior related to cancer. *Psychology and Health, 4*, 99-109.

Sheeran, P., & Orbell, S. (1996). How confidently can we infer health beliefs from questionnaire responses? *Psychology and Health, 11*, 273-290.

Stanley, M.A., & Maddux, J.E. (1986). Cognitive processes in health enhancement: Investigation of a combined protection motivation and self-efficacy model. *Basic and Applied Social Psychology, 7*(2), 101-113.

Strong, B. W., Malina, R. M., Blimkie, C. J. R., Daniels, S. R., Dishman, R. K., Gutin, B., …Trudeau, F. (2005) Evidence based physical activity for school-age youth. *The Journal of Pediatrics, 146*,732-737.

Troiano, R.P., Berrigan, D., Dodd, K.W., Masse, L.C., Tilert, T., & McDowell, M. (2008). Physical activity in the United States measured by accelerometer. *Medicine & Science in Sports & Exercise, 40*, 181-188.

Tulloch, H., Reida, R., Slovinec D'Angeloa, M., Plotnikoff, R.C., Morrina, L., Beatona, L., ... Pipe, A. (2009). Predicting short and long-term exercise intentions and behavior in patients with coronary artery disease: A test of protection motivation theory. *Psychology and Health, 24* (3), 255-269.

Wurtele S.K., & Maddux, J.E. (1987). Relative contributions of protection motivation theory components in predicting exercise intentions and behavior. *Health Psychology, 6*(5), 453-466.

Zhang, Y., & Cooke, R. (2011). Using a combined motivational and volitional intervention to promote exercise and healthy dietary behavior among undergraduates. *Diabetes Research and Clinical Practice, 95*, 215-223.

In: Physical Activity Behaviors ...
Editors: Zan Gao and Zachary Pope
ISBN: 978-1-63483-635-7

Chapter 4

USING MOTIVATIONAL AND VOLITIONAL INTERVENTIONS TO PROMOTE ADOLESCENTS' PHYSICAL ACTIVITY

***Charles C. Huang*[1,*], *Zachary Pope*[2] *and Zan Gao*[2,*]**
[1]Wayland Baptist University, Plainview, TX, US
[2]University of Minnesota-Twin Cities, Minneapolis, MN, US

ABSTRACT

This study examined the impact of two protection motivation theory-based interventions on protection motivation theory constructs, physical activity intention behavior among adolescents. Specifically, the study compared the cognitive thought processes related to protection motivation theory constructs, physical activity intention and physical activity behavior between overweight/obese and normal weight adolescents. A total of 330 junior high school students were assigned to either a control group or one of the two experimental conditions: (1) a protection motivation theory-based intervention or (2) a protection motivation theory-based intervention with an added implementation intention component. The protection motivation theory-based intervention included reading a leaflet about overweight/obesity and the effects of physical

* Dr. Charles C. Huang, CMB 1227, 1900 West 7th Street, Plainview, TX, 79072 Email: huangc@wbu.edu.
* Corresponding Author address: Dr. Zan Gao, 207 Cooke Hall, 1900 University Ave. SE, Minneapolis, MN, 55455 Email: gaoz@umn.edu.

activity on preventing this health threat. As for the protection motivation theory-based intervention with the added implementation intention component, the same leaflet was read with the added step of asking participants to plan when and where they would participate in physical activity. Participants' protection motivation theory constructs, physical activity intention and behavior were measured at three time-points over a four-week period. Repeated-measures multivariate analysis of variance found no significant main effects for either intervention on protection motivation theory constructs or physical activity intention and behavior whereas a significant main effect for weight status on protection motivation theory constructs physical activity intention and physical activity behavior was detected. Follow-up tests indicated that overweight/obese adolescents reported significantly higher perceived vulnerability and response cost, as well as lower self-efficacy, physical activity intention and physical activity behavior than normal weight adolescents. Findings indicate that, compared to the control group, the interventions were not effective in promoting adolescents' physical activity intention and behavior. Overweight/obese adolescents need to enhance their self-efficacy and reduce their perceptions of physical activity costs.

Keywords: implementation intention, overweight, physical activity intention, physical activity behavior, protection motivation

INTRODUCTION

Many studies have suggested the protection motivation theory to be useful in the prediction of health-related behaviors in physical activity interventions (Floyd, Prentice-Dunn, & Rogers, 2000; Milne, Sheeran, & Orvell, 2000; Plotnikoff & Trinh, 2010; Rogers, 1975, 1983). Protection motivation theory was originally developed in 1975 by Ronald Rogers in an attempt to explain the mechanisms behind the attitudinal and behavioral change individuals undertake when facing a real or perceived threat to their health (Rogers, 1975). In the most recent full protection motivation theory model, Rogers and his colleagues (1983, 1997) proposed that a cognitive mediating process begins once information about a health threat is received. Individuals will then engage in one of two types of responses based off cognitive appraisals of the situation: a maladaptive response and an adaptive response. When engaging in the maladaptive response, one employs a threat appraisal process. Threat appraisal is the result of an individual judging the intrinsic and extrinsic rewards associated with the unhealthy alternative (e.g., playing video games rather than completing planned exercise) as being lower than his/her perceptions of the severity of the threat and his/her perceived vulnerability to the threat. In contrast, individuals employing an adaptive response will engage in a coping appraisal. A coping appraisal results from an individual's favorable perception of response efficacy and self-efficacy when considering the perceived costs of completing the adaptive response. Most research and applications of the protection motivation theory consider the effects of five main constructs (perceived severity, perceived vulnerability, self-efficacy, response efficacy, and response cost; Lippke & Plotnikoff, 2009; Milne, Orbell, & Sheeran, 2002; Plotnikoff & Trinh, 2010; Zhang & Cooke, 2011).

Two meta-analyses (Floyd et al., 2000; Milne et al., 2000) and two systematic reviews (Norman, Boer, & Seydel, 2005; Plotnikoff et al., 2010) have summarized the findings from protection motivation theory studies across various behaviors with most studies indicating the protection motivation theory to moderately effective in predicting health-related and safety-related intentions and behaviors. Protection motivation theory has also been employed in the physical activity domain. Seven studies investigated the effects of manipulating specific protection motivation theory constructs on cognitive processes related to protection motivation theory constructs, physical activity intention, and physical activity behavior (Courneya & Hellsten, 2001; Fruin et al., 1991; Graham, Prapavessis, & Cameron, 2006; Milne et al., 2002; Stanley & Maddux, 1986; Wurtele & Maddux, 1987; Zhang et al., 2011). All studies implemented interventions to manipulate protection motivation theory constructs using motivational essays or videos. The findings of these studies indicated the interventions were generally effective in influencing subsequent cognitions and intention. However, as Milne et al., (2000) illustrated in their review, the effectiveness of these protection motivation theory-based interventions in influencing subsequent behavior was limited. Thus, further research is needed to seek the best ways of intervening with factual health education interventions to promote more favorable cognitive processes related to protection motivation theory constructs as well as physical activity intention and behavior.

Only two of the aforementioned seven studies measured the stability of the effects the interventions had on subsequent changes in cognition, intention, and behaviors via a longitudinal design. Milne et al., (2002) found that all cognitive changes induced by the health education leaflet on protection motivation theory constructs remained stable over the 2-week period after the protection motivation theory-based intervention. Further, results from a study by Graham et al., (2006) indicated that the intervention improved early exercise behavior (two weeks post-intervention), but did not improve longer term exercise behavior (four weeks post-intervention). The present study compared the effect of a protection motivation theory-based intervention and a protection motivation theory-based intervention with an added implementation intention component over a period of two and four weeks.

As discussed above, researchers have found that evidence for subsequent behavior changes related to protection motivation theory-based interventions to be limited and inconsistent (Floyd et al., 2000; Milne et al., 2000). These inconsistent findings may be explained by the model of action phases (Gollwitzer, 1993; Heckhausen, 1991) which suggests that behavior change is most likely when the individual is both motivated to act (motivational stage) and has developed strategies and plans that promote behavioral enactment (volitional stage). Gollwitzer's (1993, 1999) concept of implementation intentions is an important volitional strategy to explore the ways in which motivation is translated into action. Implementation intentions are self-regulatory strategies and simply ask participants to plan when, where, and how they will exercise. Milne et al., (2002) suggested implementation intentions used in conjunction with a protection motivation theory-based intervention to significantly increase exercise behavior over one week, compared to targeting the constructs of protection motivation theory without the use of implementation intentions. Therefore, it can be concluded that combining a protection motivation theory-based intervention with an added implementation intention component (a volitional strategy) intervention may be more effective than using a protection motivation theory-based motivational intervention only. The present study will add to the growing literature on the role of implementation intentions in health psychology by assessing their utility within the framework of protection motivation theory-based interventions.

Research suggests obesity to have far reaching effects on the health of many Americans—even among adolescents (Mokdad et al., 2003; Mokdad et al., 2004). As a result, obesity or overweight is a clear health threat to adolescents. As protection motivation theory was developed to explain health behavior motivation based on a disease prevention/health threat perspectives, it was chosen as a theoretical model in this study to explain physical activity intentions and behaviors with the objective being the prevention of obesity or overweight in this population. Although the protection motivation theory model shows promise in predicting the likelihood that individuals will adopt healthier lifestyle trends, no studies have attempted to compare the effects of manipulating protection motivation theory constructs on physical activity intention and behavior between adolescents with a health threat (i.e., overweight/obese youth) and adolescents without a health threat (i.e., normal weight youth).

Therefore, this study was designed to assess the differences among cognitions related to the protection motivation theory constructs of intention and behavior as well as the effects of a protection motivation theory-based intervention between overweight/obese and normal weight adolescents.

The purposes of this study were: (1) To investigate whether a protection motivation theory-based intervention employing a factual health education leaflet alone would change adolescents' cognitive processes related to protection motivation theory constructs, physical activity intention and physical activity behavior compared to a control; (2) To examine whether a protection motivation theory-based intervention with an added implementation intention component would change adolescents' cognitive processes related to protection motivation theory constructs, physical activity intention and physical activity behavior compared to a control and; (3) To examine the perceptual differences related to physical activity intention and behavior between overweight/obese and normal weight adolescents.

Hypotheses for purpose 1 are as follows: a). The protection motivation theory-based intervention would promote favorable cognitions related to self-efficacy, response efficacy, perceived severity, perceived vulnerability, and reduce response costs compared to the control; b). The motivational intervention would increase intention to engage in at least 60 minutes of physical activity daily over the following two weeks compared to the control; and c).

The effects of the motivational intervention on cognitive processes related to protection motivation theory constructs and PA intention will remain stable over four weeks post-intervention. Hypotheses for purpose 2 follow: The addition of an implementation intention component to the protection motivation theory-based intervention will increase adolescents' participation in at least 60 minutes of physical activity daily over two weeks compared to the conditions without any interventions and with the protection motivation theory-based intervention only. Finally, the following are hypotheses for purpose 3: a). Overweight/obese adolescents will rate their personal cognitions about the severity and personal vulnerability of the health threat higher than normal weight adolescents; and b). Overweight/obese adolescents will rate their personal self-efficacy and response efficacy lower than normal weight adolescents.

METHODS

Participants

The participating school was a suburban public school in the Mountain West Region of the United States. There were 412 seventh through ninth grade students enrolled in 12 physical education classes with class sizes ranging from 28 to 40 students with two experienced physical education teachers (one male and one female) teaching the classes. In the present study, 378 students agreed to participate in the study. The age range of the students was 11-15 years old ($Mean_{age}$ = 13.39, Standard Deviation = .97). Additional demographic information for the groups is available in Table 1.

Table 1. Demographic Distributions of Groups

			Grade			Sex	
	n	Age	7th	8th	9th	Male	Female
Group1	108	13.34±1.01	37	33	38	53	55
Group2	99	13.36±1.00	34	36	29	49	50
Group3	123	13.37±.91	43	47	33	61	62
Normal Weight	236	13.38±.97	83	86	67	121	115
Overweight/Obesity	94	13.43±.98	31	30	33	42	52
Total	330	13.39±.97	114	116	100	163	167

Note. Group1 = control group; Group 2 = motivational group; Group 3 = motivational + volitional group.

Permission to conduct the study was obtained from the University Institutional Review Board, the district, the school administration, and the physical education teachers prior to the start of this study. Students and parents provided written informed assent and consent, respectively, prior to participation in this study.

Instrumentation

Demographics. Students self-reported gender, age, grade, and race on a demographic sheet. The students' height was measured by a Seca Stadiometer

(Accurate to .1 cm; Seca Corp, CA) and weight was measured by a Taylor Digital Scale (Accurate to .1 kg, Model 7340B; Taylor Precision Products, Oak Brook, IL).

Motivational Intervention Materials. Two separate leaflets were produced for this study. The first leaflet was designed to incorporate the five major constructs of protection motivation theory: perceived severity, perceived vulnerability, response efficacy, self-efficacy, and response cost. This leaflet contained factual information about the prevalence and nature of overweight/obesity and the effects of physical activity on preventing this health threat. The content validity was confirmed by five health education specialists (two professors and three school health education teachers). All specialists agreed that the leaflet contained major relevant information and made minor revisions to the leaflet where needed. The application of all protection motivation theory constructs were modified from Milne et al., (2002) based on the condition of interest in this study (Overweight/obesity as the health threat as opposed to coronary heart disease). This first leaflet was used with Groups 2 and 3.A second leaflet was produced for the attention control condition (Group 1). It was the opening paragraphs of a novel and was in similar length to the first leaflet but had content unrelated to physical activity (King, 2011).

Implementation Intention Intervention. In addition to reading the first leaflet outlined above, Group 3 had an added implementation intention intervention component developed based on previous studies (Gollwitzer, 1993; Gollwitzer & Brandstatter, 1997; Milne et al., 2002). Students were asked to complete the following statements: "During the next 2 weeks, I will participate in at least 60 minutes of physical activity per day by ___ (physical activity(-ies)______ on_____(day or days)_____at_____(time of day) at/or in (place)_____."

Protection Motivation Theory Constructs and Intention. Measures of protection motivation theory constructs and intention (Milne et al., 2002) were employed and necessary modifications were made (obesity as the health threat instead of coronary heart disease) for this study. The measures were assessed on 5-point Likert scales, comprising belief statements coupled with appropriate response items. All the items were randomized so that patterns of questions were less obvious to the students (Sheeran & Orbell, 1996). Perceived severity was measured by one item, namely, 'If I were to develop overweight/obesity I would suffer a lot of health problems (*strongly disagree—strongly agree*).' Perceived vulnerability was measured by two items, such as, 'My chances of developing overweight/obesity in the future are (*not at all strong—very strong*).' Response efficacy was measured by one item, namely, 'Participating in physical activity at least 60 minutes daily is a good way of reducing the risk of developing overweight/obesity (strongly disagree—strongly agree).' Self-efficacy was measured by four items, such as, 'I feel confident in my ability to participate in physical activity at least 60 minutes daily in the next two weeks (*strongly agree—strongly disagree*).' Response cost was measured by four items, such as, 'The benefits of taking physical activity for 60 minutes daily outweigh the costs (*strongly agree—strongly disagree*).' Physical activity intention was measured by two items, such as, 'I do not wish to participate in physical activity at least 60 minutes daily in the next two weeks (*strongly agree—strongly disagree*).' To score each construct, the scores for items that were reverse scored were first recoded. Then, the mean score for all items for each construct were calculated. All the variables measured by multiple items formed reliable scales, with Cronbach's α values ranging from .73 to .95 (Milne et al., 2002).

Physical Activity Levels. Self-reported physical activity behavior has been shown previously to be reliable and correlated with accelerometer data in adolescents (Prochaska, Sallis, & Long, 2001). A two-item overall physical activity questionnaire (Durant et al., 2008) was employed in this study. Students were asked, 'How many days in a typical week were you physically active for at least 60 minutes?' and 'How many days in the past week were you physically active for at least 60 minutes?' Moderate reliability (intraclass coefficient= .61) has been demonstrated in adolescents aged 12-18 years (Durant et al., 2008).

Students' in-class physical activity levels were measured using ActiGraph GT1M accelerometers (Pensacola, FL). More recently, researchers demonstrated acceptable validity and reliability of the ActiGraph GT1M when used with adolescents (e.g., Corder et al., 2007). Cut points established by Freedson and colleagues (2005) were applied to the data: (a) 0–149 counts = sedentary; (b) 150–499 counts = light; and, (c) 500-3999 counts = moderate; (d) 4000-7599 counts = vigorous; (e) >7600 counts = very vigorous physical activity. In this study, students' percentage of time spent in moderate-to-vigorous physical activity was used as the outcome variable.

Body weight category. Body mass index is a measure used to determine childhood overweight and obesity in large scale studies. The Centers for Disease Control and Prevention Growth Charts (Centers for Disease Control and Prevention, 2011) were used to determine the corresponding body mass index-for-age and sex percentile. For children and adolescents (aged 2-19 years). Table 2 lists the Centers for Disease Control and Prevention cut-off points for body mass index for overweight and obesity by gender between 11 and 15 years(i.e., >85%$^{-ile}$ for age and sex).

Table 2. CDC BMI Cut-off Points for Overweight/Obesity by Gender between 11 and 15 Years

	Underweight		Overweight		Obesity	
Age	Boys	Girls	Boys	Girls	Boys	Girls
11	14.5	14.3	20.2	20.8	23.2	24.2
12	15.0	14.8	21.0	21.7	24.2	25.2
13	15.4	15.3	21.8	22.5	25.2	26.2
14	16.0	15.8	22.6	23.3	26.0	27.2
15	16.5	16.3	23.4	24.0	26.8	28.1

Procedures

During the week prior to the intervention, the principal researcher explained the basic procedures, assent form, and parental information letter to students during their respective physical education classes. At this time, the students had an opportunity to ask any questions regarding their possible participation in the study after which the students willing to participate in the study read and signed the assent form. Finally, based on students' physical education class assignment, students were randomly allocated to one of the three study groups: (1) attentional control condition: read the first three paragraphs of a book unrelated to physical activity; (2) protection motivation theory-based intervention alone: read a health education leaflet regarding the health threat of overweight and obesity and how physical activity impacts this health threat; and (3) protection motivation theory-based intervention with added implementation intention component: engaged in the same intervention as Group 2 but were also asked to outline how engaging in greater physical activity levels would be achieved in the coming weeks.

The study design was five weeks in duration and was a repeated measures factorial design involving a one week baseline measurement time period and three waves of data collection over a subsequent 4-week period following the interventions. Baseline measurements (the week prior to interventions) included the collection of participants' demographic information, physical activity intention, self-reported physical activity behavior during the previous week, and in-class physical activity levels. The details of the intervention schedule are as follows. At Time 1, participants in Group 2 and Group 3 received the motivational intervention by reading a health education leaflet, while Group 1 was asked to read the three opening paragraphs of a novel. Then, protection motivation theory constructs, physical activity intention, and in-class physical activity levels were measured among all the three groups. At Time 2, protection motivation theory constructs, physical activity intention, and in-class physical activity levels were measured again. Participants also reported their physical activity behavior in the previous week at this time. After completing the measurements, Group 3 received the implementation intention-based volitional intervention. Group 1 and Group 2 did nothing further. Finally, at Time 3, all participants again completed measures of protection motivation theory constructs, physical activity intention, self-reported physical activity behavior, and in-class physical activity levels. At this time, Group 1 received neither intervention, Group 2 (only received the protection motivation theory intervention, and Group 3 received the protection motivation theory intervention with the implementation intention component once more.

Students were taught how to wear an accelerometer by the principal researcher. All accelerometers were worn around the waist on the right hip. The distribution and collection procedures for the accelerometers were also clarified prior to data collection. Before lining up to take roll, students put on their accelerometers. During the last 5 minutes of each class, students were instructed to place their accelerometers back on top of a folder with a designated number.

Data Analysis

SPSS 18.0 Missing Values Analysis was used to highlight the patterns of missing values as well as replace them in the data set. Descriptive statistics procedures were ran to identify univariate outliers while multivariate outliers were identified using Mahalanobis distance. A one-way analysis of variance was used to check whether there were significant differences among the three groups in terms of previous physical activity level, intention, and demographics prior to the study. Differences in intention or any of the protection motivation theory constructs between Group 2 and Group 3 were also examined to determine whether the implementation intention intervention component was confounded by the differences on intentions or the variables influencing intentions. In order to check whether the interventions differentially impacted adolescents who were more and less active at baseline, cluster analysis was conducted on students' self-reported physical activity levels to determine more active students and less active students. A subsequent 3 (intervention) × 3 (time) multivariate analysis of variance was conducted to discern the interventions' effect on all study variables over time within the more active group and the less active group, respectively.

A 3 (intervention) × 2 (body weight) × 3 (time) mixed model multivariate analysis of variance with two between-subjects factors (three levels of interventions: control, protection motivation intervention along, protection motivation intervention with added implementation intention component; two levels of body weight [overweight/obesity vs. normal]) and one within-subjects factor (three levels: Time 1, Time 2, Time 3) was used to test the main effects of intervention condition, time, and body weight and the interactions of intervention × time, body weight × time, intervention × body weight, and intervention × body weight × time. Follow-up univariate tests were conducted if the multivariate analysis of variance were significant.

RESULTS

Data Entry and Screening

Initially, 378 students were recruited for the study. As a result of two students transferring to other schools and four students withdrawing from the research process, 372 students completed all measurements at all three time points. SPSS 18.0 Missing Values Analysis was used to highlight patterns of missing values finding the percentage for missing values for each variable ranged from 0% to 21.50%. Missing values were subsequently imputed by expectation maximization.

To identify any potential univariate outliers in the data set visual inspection and frequency distributions were first applied. Second, box and whisker plots, and stem-and-leaf diagrams were utilized to identify scores that appeared unattached to the bulk of the distribution. Cell values above a Z-score of 3.29 were deleted (Tabachnick & Fidell, 2007) and regarded as univariate outliers. A total of 35 cases were identified and deleted as univariate outliers following these strategies, leaving 337 cases. Additionally, seven other cases were identified through Mahalanobis distance as multivariate outliers with $p < 0.001$. After removing the seven multivariate outliers, the final sample for analysis was 330 cases (163 boys, 167 girls).

Randomization Checks and Descriptive Analysis

A one-way analysis of variance was conducted to test for any potential differences between the three groups at baseline. The results of the test revealed that there were no significant differences between the three groups in terms of previous self-reported physical activity behavior ($F(2, 327) = 1.14$, $p > 0.05$), previous intention for physical activity ($F(2, 327) = 2.33$, $p > 0.05$), students' height ($F(2, 327) = .20$, $p > 0\ .05$), students' weight ($F(2, 327) = 2.51$, $p > 0.05$), and students' age ($F(2, 327) = .18$, $p > 0.05$). However, there was a significant difference ($F(2, 327) = 12.59$, $p < 0.01$) between groups on in-class physical activity levels. Therefore, the dependent variable of in-class physical activity levels was omitted from this study. A chi-square analysis revealed no significant differences between gender ($\chi^2(2) = .01$, $p > 0.05$).

Means and standard deviations of all variables for all groups at each time point are presented in Table 3. Overall, the students strongly agreed that overweight or obesity would lead to numerous health problems, that participating in physical activity at least 60 minutes a day was a good way to reduce the risk of developing overweight/obesity, and felt confident to participate in physical activity. The students did not feel very vulnerable to develop overweight/obesity in the future and also felt the benefits of physical activity outweighed the costs. The values for physical activity intention showed that the students had high intentions to participate in physical activity. Regarding self-reported physical activity behaviors, the means suggested students to be physically active for at least 60 minutes per day for more than 4 days every week.

Students were classified into a more active group and a less active group by cluster analysis based on self-reported baseline physical activity levels. The more active group included 185 adolescents (103 boys, 82 girls) and the less active group included 145 adolescents (60 boys, 85 girls). The results of 3 (intervention) × 3 (time) multivariate analysis of variance for the more active group indicated a nonsignificant main effect for intervention on cognitive processes related to protection motivation theory constructs, physical activity intention, and physical activity behavior (Wilk's lambda = 0.89, $F(14, 352) = 1.58$, $p > 0.05$, $\eta^2 = .06$) and for the condition × time interaction (Wilk's lambda = .83, $F(28, 338) = 1.20$, $p > 0.05$, $\eta^2 = 0.09$). The multivariate analysis of variance revealed a main effect for time (Wilk's lambda = .86, $F(14, 169) = 2.05$, $p < 0.05$, $\eta^2 = 0.15$). In sum, the intervention was not effective among more active adolescents.

Table 3. Descriptive Statistics for Groups over Each Time Point

Variable	Time	Control	Motivation	Motivation +Volition	Normal Weight	Overweight/ Obesity
	T	N = 108	N = 99	N = 123	N = 236	N = 94
		M(SD)	M(SD)	M(SD)	M(SD)	M(SD)
Perceived Severity	T1	4.32(1.01)	4.33(.80)	4.50(.73)	4.45(.84)	4.24(.87)
	T2	4.16(1.12)	4.30(1.03)	4.26(1.01)	4.23(1.11)	4.28(.91)
	T3	4.33(.99)	4.17(1.18)	4.34(1.09)	4.28(1.14)	4.30(.97)
Perceived vulnerability	T1	1.95(.88)	2.20(.99)	2.19(1.00)	1.86(.86)	2.75(.92)
	T2	1.93(.90)	2.08(.95)	2.13(.96)	1.82(.88)	2.62(.83)
	T3	1.95(.98)	2.11(1.02)	2.07(.91)	1.80(.91)	2.63(.84)
Response efficacy	T1	4.54(.87)	4.66(.62)	4.66(.59)	4.68(.68)	4.48(.73)
	T2	4.72(.61)	4.61(.71)	4.72(.53)	4.71(.61)	4.63(.63)
	T3	4.55(.72)	4.39(1.02)	4.43(.97)	4.48(.95)	4.42(.82)
Self-Efficacy	T1	3.71(.96)	3.81(.86)	3.88(.82)	3.85(.89)	3.69(.84)
	T2	3.90(.89)	3.79(.85)	3.96(.85)	3.97(.88)	3.68(.80)
	T3	3.95(.93)	3.95(.92)	3.95(.82)	4.03(.90)	3.74(.80)
Response Cost	T1	2.06(.75)	1.93(.76)	1.90(.78)	1.90(.75)	2.12(.78)
	T2	1.91(.75)	2.00(.85)	1.72(.66)	1.80(.77)	2.02(.70)
	T3	1.89(.85)	1.99(.91)	1.84(.75)	1.81(.80)	2.13(.87)
Intention	T1	4.14(.93)	4.04(1.06)	4.09(.96)	4.18(.96)	3.82(.99)
	T2	4.35(.81)	4.02(.94)	4.25(.85)	4.26(.88)	4.10(.85)
	T3	4.21(.94)	4.06(1.03)	4.15(.88)	4.24(.95)	3.93(.86)
Physical Activity Behavior	T1	4.38(1.62)	4.63(1.56)	4.31(1.60)	4.61(1.53)	3.98(1.67)
	T2	4.74(1.49)	5.00(1.29)	4.63(1.42)	4.93(1.31)	4.40(1.57)
	T3	4.81(1.52)	4.93(1.24)	4.81(1.52)	5.02(1.37)	4.41(1.52)

As for the results of 3 (intervention) × 3 (time) multivariate analysis of variance for the less active group, data indicated a statistically significant main effect for intervention on cognitive processes related to protection motivation theory constructs, physical activity intention, and physical activity behavior (Wilk's lambda = 0.80, $F(14, 272) = 2.36$, $p < 0.01$, $\eta^2 = 0.11$) and for time (Wilk's lambda = .44, $F(14, 129) = 11.88$, $p < 0.01$, $\eta^2 = 0.56$).

A multivariate analysis of variance revealed a non-significant effect for the condition × time interaction (Wilk's lambda = .76, $F(28, 258) = 1.33$, $p > 0.05$, $\eta^2 = 0.13$).

Further pairwise comparisons revealed differences to only exist between Group 2 and Group 3 on the protection motivation theory construct of perceived severity ($p < 0.05$). Given these data, the intervention was also not effective among less active adolescents.

Effect of Interventions on Protection Motivation Theory Constructs and Intention

The main hypotheses were tested by conducting a mixed model multivariate analysis of variance with two between-subject factors (3 levels of intervention conditions and 2 levels of weight conditions) and one within-subjects factor (3 levels time). multivariate analysis of variance yielded a nonsignificant main effect for intervention condition on protection motivation theory constructs and intention (Wilk's lambda = 0.94, $F(12, 638) = 1.54$, $p > 0.05$, $\eta^2 = 0.03$), the condition × time interaction (Wilk's lambda = 0.90, $F(24, 626) = 1.35$, $p > 0.05$, $\eta^2 = 0.05$), the condition × time × weight category interaction (Wilk's lambda = 0.90, $F(24, 626) = 1.41$, $p > 0.05$, $\eta^2 = 0.05$), and the time × weight category (Wilk's lambda = 0.96, $F(12, 313) = 1.15$, $p > 0.05$, $\eta^2 = 0.04$). multivariate analysis of variance did reveal a main effect for time (Wilk's lambda = 0.87, $F(12, 312) = 4.05$, $p < 0.001$, $\eta^2 = 0.13$). However, because the interaction of condition × time was not statistically significant, the changes among protection motivation theory constructs and physical activity intention over time were parallel between groups. Therefore, this time effect was not produced by the intervention.

The results suggested that neither of the two protection motivation theory-based interventions successfully impacted the protection motivation theory constructs or physical activity intention. As such, the hypotheses (a) and (b) for purpose 1 were not supported by the results.

Additionally, the third hypothesis, which stated the effect of the intervention on protection motivation theory constructs and physical activity intention would remain stable over the 4-week study duration, was not tested because of the non-significant main effect for intervention condition.

Effect of Interventions on Physical Activity Behavior

A multivariate analysis of variance revealed a non-significant main effect for the intervention condition on self-reported physical activity behavior ($F(2, 324) = 2.36$, $p > 0.05$, $\eta^2 = 0.02$) as well as the condition × time interaction (Wilk's lambda = 0.99, $F(4, 646) = .63$, $p > 0.05$, $\eta^2 = 0.01$). A significant main effect for time (Wilk's lambda = 0.93, $F(2, 323) = 12.72$, $p < 0.001$, $\eta^2 = 0.07$) was detected. Similar to the above section, because the interaction of condition × time was not statistically significant, the changes of physical activity behavior over time were parallel between groups. Therefore, the time effect was not produced by the intervention. The findings suggested that the interventions did not promote participants' physical activity behavior and, thus, the hypothesis for purpose 2 was not supported. Specifically, the addition of an implementation intention component to the protection motivation theory-based intervention did not further increase adolescents' participation in at least 60 minutes of PA per day during the 2 weeks after the intervention.

Body Weight Group Differences of Protection Motivation Theory Constructs, Intention, and Behavior

A multivariate analysis of variance indicated a significant effect for body weight categories on cognitive processes related to protection motivation theory constructs and intentions (Wilk's lambda = .78, $F(6, 318) = 14.76$, $p < 0.01$, $\eta^2 = 0.22$), and self-reported physical activity behaviors ($F(1, 324) = 17.71$, $p < .01$, $\eta^2 = 0.05$). Follow-up tests revealed that there were statistically significant differences between overweight/obese participants and normal weight participants on perceived vulnerability, self-efficacy, response cost, intention, and self-reported physical activity behavior (See Table 4). In detail, overweight/obese participants reported higher perceived vulnerability and response cost than normal weight participants. They also reported significantly lower self-efficacy, intention, and physical activity behavior. These findings partially support the hypotheses for purpose 3. Specifically, overweight/obese adolescents rated their personal beliefs about the severity and personal vulnerability to the threat of obesity as higher than normal weight adolescents—although only personal vulnerability was statistically different. Second, overweight/obese adolescents rated their personal self-efficacy and response-efficacy lower than normal weight adolescents, but only self-efficacy was statistically lower.

Table 4. Protection Motivation Theory Constructs, Intention and Behavior Means Across Body Weight Groups

Variable	Normal Weight *M(SD)*	Overweight & Obesity *M(SD)*	F	*p*	η^2
Perceived Severity	4.32(.05)	4.22(.09)	.837	.364	.003
Perceived Vulnerability	1.83(.05)**	2.67(.08)**	87.97	.000	.214
Response Efficacy	4.62(.04)	4.51(.06)	2.34	.127	.007
Self-Efficacy	3.95(.05)**	3.68(.07)**	9.32	.002	.028
Response Cost	1.85(.04)**	2.10(.07)**	9.37	.002	.028
Intention	4.22(.05)**	3.96(.08)**	7.68	.006	.023
Behavior	4.86(.08)**	4.21(.13)**	17.71	.000	.052

Note. ** significant difference between groups at $p < .01$.

DISCUSSION

Effect of Interventions on Protection Motivation Theory Constructs and Intention

Findings revealed no significant effects for the protection motivation theory-based interventions with regard to changing cognitive processes related to protection motivation theory constructs or physical activity intention. Therefore, the hypotheses that the interventions would increase self-efficacy, response efficacy, perceived severity, perceived vulnerability, and reduce response costs compared to the control condition, in addition to the hypothesis that the interventions would increase intention to engage in 60 or more minutes of physical activity per day over the following two weeks after the intervention compared to the control condition, were not supported. These results are inconsistent with Milne et al., (2002) and Zhang et al., (2011). Milne et al., (2002) conducted a study on a protection motivation theory-based intervention among 248 undergraduate students and reported the intervention had a significant impact on the cognitive processes related to protection motivation theory constructs and exercise intentions, but not on physical activity behavior, in a 1-week follow-up. Zhang et al., (2011) also conducted a protection motivation theory-based health education intervention among undergraduate students reporting the intervention had significant positive effects on the cognitive processes related to protection motivation theory constructs and exercise intentions.

There are several potential reasons for the inconsistency between the present study and past literature. First, this is the first study to use overweight/obesity as a health threat in the application of protection motivation theory. Previous studies used colon cancer (Courneya & Hellsten, 2001; Graham et al., 2006), coronary heart disease (Milne et al., 2002), and diabetes (Zhang et al., 2012) as the health threat source for the intervention. As a result, this factor might have influenced the effects the intervention had on protection motivation theory constructs and intention. Specifically, protection motivation theory proposes that if communication of health threat information evokes fear, then the recipient will be motivated to reduce this unpleasant emotional state and modify associated behaviors. Overweight/obesity might not evoke equivalent amounts of fear in comparison to other diseases (e.g., colon cancer, coronary heart disease, and diabetes) leading to discrepancies between the findings of the current study and previous studies. Comparisons of the means of protection motivation theory constructs in this study to those of previous studies reveals the students in the present study perceived lower vulnerability than those in previous studies. Means of perceived vulnerability to overweight or obesity among each group at different time-points ranged from 1.95 to 2.20 (39% to 44% on the 5-point scale) in this study. However, participants in a study conducted by Graham et al., (2006) reported the perceived vulnerability to colon cancer to range from 3.53 to 4.32 (50% to 62% on a 7-point scale). Similarly, in a study conducted by Milne et al., (2002), participants' perceived vulnerability to coronary heart disease among each group at every time-point ranged from 3.86 to 4.44 (55% to 63% on a 7-point scale) while Zhang et al., (2012) reported participants' perceived vulnerability to diabetes ranged from 2.43 to 3.91 (49% to 78% on a 5-point scale). Therefore, the relatively lower perceived vulnerability in this study might suggest that students did not feel particularly vulnerable to the threat of overweight/obesity. Further, these lower perceived vulnerability scores might partially explain the nonsignificant effect of the intervention on physical activity intention.

A second factor contributing to the inconsistency might be age. Previous studies recruited college students (Milne et al., 2002; Zhang et al., 2011), physically inactive teaching and school staff (Graham et al., 2006), and adults between the ages of 18 and 65 years (Plotnikoff et al., 2009). Only one study

(Fruin et al., 1991) recruited adolescents and, specifically, 9th and 10th grade high school students. However, participants in this study were 7th to 9th grade junior high school students (11 to 15 years old). According to Piaget's theory of cognitive development (Bjorklund, 2004), children's thought processes are oriented to things and events that they can observe directly, whereas adolescents can think more hypothetically and abstractly. Students in the present study are transitioning from childhood to adolescence. Thus, the limitations in abstract thinking may become a hindrance to the cognitive processes related to health threats and intention to change behavior if the student was not already experiencing overweight/obesity.

Third, students' prior knowledge about the intervention materials might be another factor contributing to the non-significant effects of the interventions. After reading the leaflet serving as the protection motivation theory-based intervention material, students were asked to rate their mastery of information on the leaflet. The information included the prevalence and nature of overweight or obesity, and the effects of physical activity on preventing this health threat. The mean was 3.51 (5-point scale) with a standard deviation of 0.95. These findings suggest that students in this study had mastered about 70% of the information presented in the intervention leaflet. After reviewing 183 published books, articles, papers, and research reports, Dochy, Segers, and Buehl (1999) concluded that prior knowledge was strongly associated with the construction of new conceptions or perceptions. Thus, the relatively higher mastery of prior knowledge (70%) in this study might result in relatively higher scores on perceived severity, self-efficacy, response efficacy, intention, and might have led to relatively lower scores on response costs and perceived vulnerability for all groups (See Table 3). Finally, considerably high or low scores might have produced ceiling or floor effects, respectively (Lammers & Badia, 2005) and masked the potential effect of the interventions.

Milne et al., (2002) found that the protection motivation theory-based intervention significantly improved the cognitive processes related to protection motivation theory constructs and exercise intentions. Moreover, all these cognitive changes induced by the intervention on protection motivation theory constructs and intention remained stable over a 2-week period. However, whether the effects of the intervention on protection motivation theory constructs and physical activity intention remained stable over the 4-week duration of the present study was not examined due to the fact the intervention did not significantly impact the students' cognitive processes related to protection motivation theory constructs and physical activity intention. Further, this stability was not examined given the significant main effect for time (Wilk's lambda = 0.87, $F(12, 312) = 4.05$, $p < 0.001$, $\eta^2 = 0.13$) suggesting the cognitive processes related to protection motivation theory constructs and physical activity intention changed over time. This time effect was not produced by the intervention, however, as the interaction of condition × time was not significant.

Effect of Interventions on Physical Activity Behavior

There were no significant main effects for intervention conditions on students' self-reported physical activity behavior or a significant interaction of condition × time. This implies that the interventions did not effectively promote the students' physical activity behavior. Thus, the research hypothesis was not supported. This was consistent with the study conducted by Milne et al., (2002) who reported a protection motivation theory-based intervention among undergraduate students had a significant impact on physical activity intentions but not on physical activity behavior in during the 1-week follow-up. However, in a similar protection motivation theory-based intervention among undergraduate students, Zhang et al., (2011) reported the intervention had significant positive effects on protection motivation theory constructs, physical activity intentions, and physical activity behavior. In line with Zhang et al.'s positive findings, Graham et al., (2006) examined whether colon cancer was a meaningful source of exercise motivation finding an intervention effect in exercise behavior at two weeks postintervention—although these effects were not seen at four weeks postintervention. These inconsistent results suggest further studies should be conducted on the effects of protection motivation theory-based interventions in relation to physical activity behavior.

Conversely, a large body of published experimental studies have suggested that implementation intention interventions were successful in changing physical activity behavior (Armitage & Sorigg, 2010; Kwak, Kremers, Van Baak, & Brug, 2007; Luszczynska & Haynes, 2009; Milne et al., 2002; Prestwich, Perugini, & Hurling, 2010; Roberts, Maddison, Magnusson, & Prapavessis, 2010; Scholz, Knoll, Sniehotta, & Schwarzer, 2006; Sniehotta, Scholz, & Schwarzer, 2006; Zhang et al., 2012). Despite this wealth of empirical evidence, the protection motivation theory-based intervention with the added implementation intention component did not significantly promote adolescents' physical activity behavior in this study. This was evidenced by the lack of a non-significant main effect for intervention conditions on students' self-reported physical activity behavior as well as the condition × time interaction. Although there was a significant main effect for time, it was not produced by the intervention as indicated by non-significant condition × time interaction. The inconsistent findings of the current study compared to previous studies might again be traced to the inclusion of adolescent participants in the present study versus the use of various adult populations in previous studies.

Body Weight Group Differences of Protection Motivation Theory Constructs, Intention, and Behavior

The results of the study indicated that overweight/obese participants reported higher perceptions of vulnerability and response cost than normal weight participants. Overweight/obese participants also reported significantly lower self-efficacy, physical activity intention, and physical activity behavior (see Table 4). Therefore, the hypotheses that overweight/obese adolescents would rate their personal beliefs about the severity of the threat and personal vulnerability to the threat as higher and would rate personal self-efficacy and response efficacy lower than normal weight adolescents were partially supported. Although previous studies examined perceptions of protection motivation theory constructs, intention, and physical activity behavior separately among populations with a health threat and without a health threat after interventions, no study compared perceptions of protection motivation theory constructs, intention, and behavior between populations with and without a health threat within a single study after receiving the same intervention. For example, Zhang et al., (2012) tested the impact of combining a protection motivation theory-based intervention with an added implementation intention component on protection motivation theory constructs, intention, and exercise behavior. Participants were undergraduates who did not have a history of diabetes (targeted health threat).

To our knowledge, there has been no previous study that compared perceptions of protection motivation theory constructs, physical activity intention, and physical activity behavior between overweight/obese adolescents and normal weight adolescents. The results of present study suggest adolescents with the targeted health problem have different cognitive processes related to protection motivation theory constructs, physical activity intention, and physical activity behavior versus adolescents without the targeted health problem. Specifically, compared to normal weight adolescents, overweight/obese adolescents tend to perceive that they are more likely to suffer from the health threat if they do not participate in physical activity. They also feel that participating in physical activity will cost more than normal weight adolescents. It was also implicated that overweight/obese adolescents have lower confidence to engage in physical activity than normal weight adolescents (i.e., lower self-efficacy scores). As such, physical activity interventions for overweight/obese adolescents should focus on changing perceived vulnerability to the health threat, self-efficacy for physical activity, and the perceived physical activity costs.

In conclusion, the current protection motivation theory-based intervention failed to change adolescents' cognitive processes related to protection motivation theory constructs, physical activity intention, and physical activity behavior. Further, adding an implementation intention component to the protection motivation theory-based intervention was also not effective enough to promote adolescents' physical activity behavior.

Overweight/obese adolescents perceived different levels of most of the protection motivation theory constructs, physical activity intention, and physical activity behavior compared to the normal weight adolescents. Specifically, overweight/obese adolescents felt more likely to be overweight/obese if they did not change their physical activity behavior and that it costs more to participate in physical activity compared to normal weight adolescents. Overweight/obese adolescents have lower confidence to engage in physical activity than normal weight adolescents. Their physical activity levels and intention to participate in physical activity were also lower than normal weight adolescents.' Yet, despite the fact overweight/obese adolescents had different perceptions, they did not respond to either intervention differently than normal weight adolescents.

References

Armitage, C.J., & Sprigg, C.A. (2010). The roles of behavioral and implementation intentions in changing physical activity in young children with low socioeconomic status. *Journal of Sport and Exercise Psychology, 32*, 359-376.

Bjorklund, D.F. (2004). *Children's thinking: Cognitive development and individual differences.* Stamford, CT: Wadsworth Publishing.

Blanchard, C.M., Reid, R.D., Morrin, L.I., McDonnell, L., McGannon, K., Rhodes, R.E., … Edwards, N. (2009). Does protection motivation theory explain exercise intentions and behavior during home-based cardiac rehabilitation? *Journal of Cardiopulmonary Rehabilitation & Prevention, 29*(3), 188-192.

Centers for Disease Control and Prevention. (2011). About BMI for children and teens, Retrieved from http://www.cdc.gov/healthyweight/assessing/bmi/childrens_bmi/about_childrens_bmi.html.

Corder, K., Brage, S., Ramachandran, A., Snehalatha, C., Wareham, N., & Ekelund, U. (2007). Comparison of two Actigraph models for assessing free-living physical activity in Indian adolescents. *Journal of Sports Sciences, 25*, 1607–1611.

Courneya, K.S., & Hellsten, L.A.M. (2001). Cancer prevention as a source of exercise motivation: An experimental test using protection motivation theory. *Psychology, Health and Medicine, 6*(1), 59-64.

Dochy, F., Segers, M., & Buehal, M.M. (1999). The relation between assessment practices and outcomes of studies: The case of research on prior knowledge. *Review of Educational Research, 69*, 145-186.

Durant, N., Harris, S.K., Doyle, S., Person, S., Saelens, B.E., Kerr, J., … Sallis, J.F. (2008). Relation of school environment and policy to adolescent physical activity. *Journal of School Health, 79*, 153-159.

Floyd, D.L., Prentice-Dunn, S., & Rogers, R.W. (2000). A meta-analysis of research on protection motivation theory. *Journal of Applied Social Psychology, 30*(2), 407-429.

Freedson, P., Pober, D., & Janz, K.F. (2005). Calibration of accelerometer output for children. *Medicine & Science in Sports & Exercise, 37*(11), S523-S530.

Fruin, D.J., Pratt, C., & Owen, N. (1991). Protection motivation theory and adolescents' perceptions of exercise. *Journal of Applied Social Psychology, 22*(1), 55-69.

Gollwitzer, P.M. (1993). Goal achievement: The role of intentions. *European Review of Social Psychology, 4*, 141-185.

Gollwitzer, P.M. (1999). Implementation intentions: Strong effects of simple plans. *American Psychologist, 54*, 493-503.

Gollwitzer, P.M., & Brandstatter, V. (1997). Implementation intentions and effective goal pursuit. *Journal of Personality and Social Psychology, 73*, 186-199.

Graham, S.P., Prapavessis, H., & Cameron, L.D. (2006). Colon cancer information as a source of exercise motivation. *Psychology and Health, 21*(6), 739-755.

Heckhausen, H. (1991). *Motivation and action.* New York, NY: Springer.

King, A.S. (2011). *Everybody sees the ants.* New York, NY: Little, Brown and Company.

Kwak, L., Kremers, S.P.J., Van Baak, M., & Brug, J. (2007). Formation of implementation intentions promote stair use. *American Journal of Preventive Medicine, 32*, 254-255.

Lammers, W.J., & Badia, P. (2005). *Fundamental of behavioral research.* Belmont, CA: Thomson and Wadsworth.

Lippke, S., & Plotnikoff, R.C. (2009). The protection motivation theory within the stages of the transtheoretical model – State-specific interplay of variables and prediction of exercise stage transitions. *British Journal of Health Psychology, 14*, 211-229.

Luszczynska, A., & Haynes, C. (2009). Changing nutrition, physical activity and body weight among student nurses and midwives: Effects of a planning intervention and self-efficacy beliefs. *Journal of Health Psychology, 14*, 1075-1084.

Milne, S., Orbell, S., & Sheeran, P. (2002). Combining motivational and volitional interventions to promote exercise participation: Protection motivation theory and implementation intentions. *British Journal of Health Psychology, 7*, 163-184.

Milne, S., Sheeran, P., & Orbell, S. (2000). Prediction and intervention in health-related behavior: A meta-analytic review of protection motivation theory. *Journal of Applied Social Psychology, 30*(1), 106-143.

Mokdad, A.H., Ford, E.S., Bowman, B.A., Dietz, W.H., Vinicor, F., Bales, V.S., & Marks, J.S. (2003). Prevalence of obesity, diabetes, and obesity-related health risk factors, 2001. *The Journal of American Medical Association, 289*(1), 76-79.

Mokdad, A.H., Marks, J.S., Stroup, D.F., & Gerberding, J.L. (2004). Actual causes of death in the United States, 2000. *The Journal of American Medical Association, 291*(10), 1238-1245.

Norman, P., Boer, H., & Seydel, E. (2005). Protection motivation theory. In M. Conner, & P. Norman (Eds.), *Predicting health behavior: Research and practice with social cognition models* (2nd ed.; pp 81-126). London: Open University Press.

Orbell, S., Hodgkins, S., & Sheeran, P. (1997). Implementation intentions and the theory of planned behavior. *Personality and Social Psychology Bulletin, 33*, 209-217.

Plotnikoff, R.C., Rhodes, R.E., & Trinh, L. (2009). Protection motivation theory: A longitudinal test among a representative population sample of Canadian adults. *Journal of Health Psychology, 14* (8), 1119-1134.

Plotnikoff, R.C., & Trinh, L. (2010). Protection motivation theory: Is this a worthwhile theory for physical activity promotion? *Exercise and Sport Sciences Reviews, 38*(2), 91-98.

Prestwich, A., Perugini, M., & Hurling, R. (2010). Can implementation intentions and text messages promote brisk walking? A randomized trial. *Health Psychology: Official Journal of the Division of Health Psychology, American Psychological Association, 29*, 40-49.

Prochaska, J.J., Sallis, J.F., & Long, B. (2001). A physical activity screening measure for use with adolescents in primary care. *Archives of Pediatrics & Adolescent Medicine, 155*(5), 554-559.

Roberts, V., Maddison, R., Magnusson, J., & Prapavessis, H. (2010). Adolescent physical activity: Does implementation intention have a role? *Journal of Physical Activity and Health, 7*, 497-507.

Rogers, R.W. (1975). A protection motivation theory of fear appeals and attitude change. *Journal of Psychology, 91*(1), 93-114.

Rogers, R.W. (1983). Cognitive and physiological processes in fear-based attitude change: A revised theory of protection motivation. In J. Cacioppo & R. Petty (Eds.), *Social psychophysiology: A sourcebook* (pp. 153-176). New York, NY: Guilford.

Rogers, R.W., & Prentice-Dunn, S. (1997). Protection motivation theory. In D. Gochman (Ed.), *Handbook of health behavior research 1: Personal and social determinants* (pp. 113-132). New York, NY: Plenum.

Scholz, U., Knoll, N., Sniehotta, F.F., & Schwarzer, R. (2006). Physical activity and depressive symptoms in cardiac rehabilitation: Long-term effects of a self-management intervention. *Social Science & Medicine, 62*, 3109-3120.

Sheeran, P., & Orbell, S. (1996). How confidently can we infer health beliefs from questionnaire responses? *Psychology and Health, 11*, 273-290.

Sniehotta, F.F., Scholz, U., & Schwarzer, R. (2006). Action plans and coping plans for physical exercise: A longitudinal intervention study in cardiac rehabilitation. *British Journal of Health Psychology, 11*, 23-37.

Stanley, M.A., & Maddux, J.E. (1986). Cognitive processes in health enhancement: Investigation of a combined protection motivation and self-efficacy model. *Basic and Applied Social Psychology, 7*(2), 101-113.

Tabachnick, B., & Fidell, L. (2007). *Using multivariate statistics* (5th ed.). Boston, MA: Person Education.

Tulloch, H., Reida, R., Slovinec D'Angeloa, M., Plotnikoff, R.C., Morrina, L., Beatona, L., ... Pipe, A. (2009). Predicting short and long-term exercise intentions and behavior in patients with coronary artery disease: A test of protection motivation theory. *Psychology and Health, 24* (3), 255-269.

Wurtele S.K., & Maddux, J.E. (1987). Relative contributions of protection motivation theory components in predicting exercise intentions and behavior. *Health Psychology, 6*(5), 453-466.

Zhang, Y., & Cooke, R. (2011). Using a combined motivational and volitional intervention to promote exercise and healthy dietary behavior among undergraduates. *Diabetes Research and Clinical Practice, 95*, 215-223.

In: Physical Activity Behaviors …
Editors: Zan Gao and Zachary Pope
ISBN: 978-1-63483-635-7

Chapter 5

ASSOCIATIONS AMONG ELEMENTARY SCHOOL CHILDREN'S SELF-EFFICACY, ENJOYMENT, AND PERCEIVED EXERTION IN EXERGAMING

Peng Zhang[1,*], Zachary Pope[2] and Zan Gao[2,*]
[1]East Stroudsburg University, East Stroudsburg, PA, US
[2]University of Minnesota-Twin Cities, Minneapolis, MN, US

ABSTRACT

This study examined the relationships among elementary school children's self-efficacy, enjoyment, and perceived exertion in a school-based exergaming program. A total of 219 third through fifth grade students responded to a battery of standardized questionnaires measuring their self-efficacy, enjoyment and rating of perceived exertion during exergaming. Correlation analyses indicated children's self-efficacy, enjoyment, and rating of perceived exertion were positively related to one another. Regression analysis further revealed that self-efficacy was a significant positive predictor for rating of perceived exertion ($\beta = .21$, $p < 0.01$). A two-way (Grade × Gender) multivariate analysis of variance

* Dr. Peng Zhang, 210 Zimbar-Liljenstein Hall, 1236 Centre St., East Stroudsburg, PA, 18301 Email pzhang@esu.edu.

* Corresponding Author address: Dr. Zan Gao, 207 Cooke Hall, 1900 University Ave. SE, Minneapolis, MN, 55455 Email: gaoz@umn.edu.

revealed that fifth grade students reported significantly lower perceived exertion ratings than third and fourth grade students, $F(2, 213) = 4.56$, $p < 0.01$. No gender differences were observed. Findings suggest children with high confidence in playing exergaming were more likely to engage and exert effort in this activity. In addition, older children might perceive exergaming as a light-intensity physical activity.

Keywords: physical activity, Dance Dance Revolution, Wii

INTRODUCTION

A high rate of inactivity is a risk factor for obesity among children and adolescents. In the U.S., less than 15% of children and adolescents participate regularly in physical activity (O'Loughlin, Dugas, Sabiston, & O'Loughlin, 2012). In fact, school children spend two to four and half hours per day watching TV and playing computer and video games (Vandewater et al., 2007). Besides the rising risk of obesity, research indicates that inactivity among children may also be associated with diabetes, cardiovascular diseases, and low self-esteem (Donnelly et al., 1996; U.S. Department of Health and Human Services, 2006).

Authorities recommend that children should participate in moderate to vigorous physical activity to reduce these health risks and increase life expectancy. For instance, the National Association for Sport and Physical Education (2009) and the National Institutes of Health (2010) recommend 60 minutes of moderate intensity physical activity daily for children and youth. The American Heart Association (2011) advocates for the same recommendations adding that the daily physical activity for children should be fun, enjoyable, and developmentally appropriate. All these recommendations emphasize the significance of regular physical activity participation among children. They also provided guidance for innovative interventions to prevent and control the childhood obesity epidemic in the U.S.

Exergaming, an innovative activity combining technology, gaming, and body movement, has the potential to promote physical activity participation among children and youth (Epstein, Paluch, Roemmich, & Beecher, 2007; Gao, Huang, Liu, & Xiong, 2012). Further, exergaming has been defined as fun, safe, and convenient interactive video games suitable for individuals of all ages (Lanningham-Foster et al., 2009). As such, health professionals have viewed exergaming as a good alternative to traditional sports and physical activities for children in the U.S. (Bailey & McInnis, 2011; Epstein et al., 2007; Gao et al., 2012; Gao, Zhang, & Stodden, 2013). Meanwhile, increasing evidence shows that K-12 teachers have integrated exergaming such as Dance Dance Revolution and Wii Fit, into their curricula (Gao, Hannon, Newton, & Huang, 2011).

In the past decade, research has shown that exergaming can have a positive influence on children's energy expenditure (Bosch, Poloni, Thorton, & Lynskey, 2012; Devereaux et al., 2012; Gao, Podlog, & Huang, 2013).

For example, in a systematic review of the exergaming literature, Gao and Chen (2014) reported that exergaming led to a light to moderate level of physical activity among children and youth. Moreover, exergaming has been recommended as a viable replacement for sedentary behaviors. However, there is a lack of consistent evidence in relation to the effectiveness of school-based exergaming on children's health outcomes (Bailey & McInnis, 2011; Fogel, Miltenberger, Graves, & Koehler, 2010; Gao & Chen, 2014). Additionally, while age-related declines in physical activity are evident in children and adolescents (Sallis, Prochaska, & Taylor, 2000), no known study has specifically addressed the age and gender differences on energy expenditure in exergaming among children. This study was designed to address the aforementioned topics.

As is well known, both self-efficacy and enjoyment have been identified as determinants of physical activity behaviors and might operate together to impact individuals' physical activity (Liang, Motl, McAuley, & Konopack, 2007). According to the social cognitive theory, self-efficacy refers to beliefs about one's capabilities to learn or perform behaviors of various difficulties (Bandura, 1997).

Substantial evidence supports the idea that self-efficacy serves as a determinant in predicting exercise adherence, persistence through challenges, and physical activity intensity levels (Gao et al., 2012; Gao, Newton, & Carson, 2008; Malherbe, Steel, & Theron, 2003; Motl et al., 2002; Ning, Gao, & Lodewyk, 2012).

Given the fact self-efficacy is regarded as situation-specific beliefs in ability (Bandura, 1997; Gao, Lochbaum, & Podlog, 2011), literature has evidenced that stronger self-efficacy leads to better performances in multiple activities, including bowling, gymnastics, bench press, and after-school physical activity (Boyce & Bingham, 1997; Fitzsimmons, Landers, Thomas, van der Mars, 1991; McAuley, 1985).

Enjoyment is also an important determinant of physical activity, and is defined as a positive psychological state characterized by a sense of fun, liking, and pleasure. Coulter and Woods (2011) reported that interventions designed to enhance, among other things, perceptions of enjoyment resulted in maintained and increased physical activity levels in children - results similar to that of Dishman et al., (2005). Research has also suggested that children and adolescents enjoy interacting with screen-based media (Epstein et al., 2007). For example, Graves and colleagues (2010) reported the Wii Fit appeared to be an enjoyable exergame for both adolescents. Thus, integrating exergaming into the school curriculum may aid in advancing the teaching objectives in physical education.

Finally, numerous literature has used the rating of perceived exertion scale as a subjective form of measurement for exercise intensity during various physical activities such as cycling, soccer, swimming, and walking (Couture, Jerome, & Tihanyi, 1999; Impellizzeri, Rampinini, & Marcora, 2005; Vuillerme & Hintzy, 2007; Wergel-Kolmert & Wohlfart, 1999).

In the last decade, researchers have also used the scale to assess individuals' perceived energy expenditure when playing exergames including Dance Dance Revolution, Wii Sports, and Wii FIT (Graves et al., 2010; Mullins, Tessmer, McCarroll, & Peppel, 2012). Pollock and colleagues found that rating of perceived exertion scale scores were positively associated with heart rate in adults during exercise sessions using the Wii FIT Plus (Pollock et al., 2012).

Knowing the correlation between children's psychological beliefs and rating of perceived exertion is an important prerequisite in designing effective intervention programs to promote physical activity in children. However, no study has investigated the relationships between elementary school children's self-efficacy, enjoyment, and ratings of perceived exertion during exergaming. Therefore, the purposes of the study were to: 1) examine the relationships between children's self-efficacy, enjoyment and ratings of perceived exertion in an exergaming program; and 2) surmise whether or not grade and gender differences exist for these outcomes. Based on the literature review, it was hypothesized that: 1) children's self-efficacy and enjoyment toward exergaming would be positively related to and would predict their ratings of perceived exertion during exergaming; 2) boys would demonstrate higher levels of self-efficacy, enjoyment, and ratings of perceived exertion for exergaming than girls; and 3) younger children would report higher levels of self-efficacy, enjoyment, and ratings of perceived exertion for exergaming than older children.

METHODS

Participants

Participants were 346 third through fifth grade children (195 boys, 151 girls) enrolled in a suburban Title I elementary school in Western Texas. The breakdown by grade was: 127 third grade students, 111 fourth grade students, 106 fifth grade students, and 2 undeclared. Children attended 150-minutes of weekly structured physical activity programs at school (two 50-minute physical education programs plus one 50-minute exergaming session) and a daily 20-minute recess after lunch. These programs were attended as a class unit with class sizes ranging from 18 to 24 children. The specific inclusion criteria for this study were: (1) children aged 8-12 years; (2) no diagnosis of a physical or mental disability according to school records; and (3) parental consent and child assent was provided. Children in these samples were selected because: (1) the age range is a critical period for children to develop and maintain a physically active lifestyle; and (2) children aged 8 years and older are able to understand and play exergames. Approval from the University Institutional Review Board and the school district were obtained. Parental consent and child assent were obtained before data collection.

Twelve exergaming stations were set up in a large classroom, with each station being equipped with various exergames including Dance Dance Revolution, Wii Just Dance, Wii Fit, and Wii Sports. A trained physical education teacher supervised the children during exergaming. Each station accommodated up to two children and children rotated from one station to another station every 15 minutes. In this manner, all children in one class had the opportunity to play exergaming simultaneously and were able to play different exergames during the program.

Instrumentation

Self-efficacy. To measure children's self-efficacy, three items were adopted from a valid and reliable measure developed by Gao and his colleagues (2012). Specifically, in this study, children responded to the items using a five-point Likert-type scale (1 = *strongly disagree*, 5 = *strongly agree*), with the stem "With regard to the exergaming, I have confidence in…" The answers were: (a) my ability to doing well in exergaming; (b) my ability to learn skills well in exergaming; and (c) my performance in exergaming. The mean of these items was used as a measure of children's self-efficacy.

Enjoyment. Enjoyment was measured using a valid and reliable assessment instrument used by Gao et al., (2012). Five items were used to assess children's enjoyment in exergaming with children responding on the same five-point Likert scale as that of self-efficacy. The five items were: (a) I have more fun playing exergaming than doing other things; (b) Playing exergaming is the thing I like to do best; (c) I wish I could play more exergaming than I get chance to; (d) I usually prefer to watch rather than play exergaming; and (e) I really like playing exergaming at school. The instrument was originally validated by Ommundsen and his associates (Ommundsen, Page, Ku, & Cooper, 2008).

Rating of Perceived Exertion. Borg's Rating of Perceived Exertion scale (Borg, 1973), a psycho-physiological measure estimating the intensity of physical effort perceived by an individual during cardiovascular or resistance training, was utilized to measure the children's perception of energy expenditure. Rating of perceived exertion includes 15 category scales, ranging from six to 20, representing eight levels of exercise intensity/efforts: no exertion at all (6), extremely light (7 - 8), very light (9 - 10), light (11 - 12), somewhat hard (13 - 14), hard or heavy (15 - 16), extremely hard (19), and maximal exertion (20).

The rating of perceived exertion scale has been validated using heart rate, different measures of ventilatory drive (i.e., oxygen uptake [VO_2], % maximal O_2 uptake [% VO_2 max] respiration rate), and blood and muscle lactate concentrations (Chen, Fan, & Moe, 2002). Skatrud-Mickelson and colleagues (2011) reported that the scale has been shown to be accurate and reliable (r = .80 - .90) in most populations in the measurement of exercise intensity while walking. Overall, through a large body of experimental evidence, the 15-point scale has proven to be a useful measure for most individuals in assessing intensity of physical activity immediately following activity (Dishman, 1994).

Procedures

Children's self-efficacy, enjoyment and ratings of perceived exertion during exergaming were measured at the end of the school year. Two research assistants were trained to assist with instructions and the data collection of the questionnaires. The children completed the survey in the exergaming gym at the end of the class. To minimize children's tendency to give socially desirable responses, children were encouraged to answer truthfully and were assured that their responses were confidential and would not affect their grades. Further, the researchers clearly stated that there was no right or wrong answers and that the physical education teachers would not have access to their responses. Finally, the researchers monitored and helped children by answering any questions they had.

DATA ANALYSES

Data were analyzed in four steps. First, the researchers calculated Cronbach's alpha coefficients to ensure the internal consistency of the self-reported questionnaires. Children's mean scores for self-efficacy, enjoyment, and ratings of perceived exertion were then calculated. Second, Pearson product moment correlations were calculated to evaluate the relationships among children's self-efficacy, enjoyment, and rating of perceived exertion during exergaming. Third, multiple regression analysis was used to determine whether children's self-efficacy and enjoyment predicted rating of perceived exertion. The last step involved performing a 2 (gender of child) × 3 (grade level) multivariate analysis of variance with self-efficacy, enjoyment, and rating of perceived exertion as dependent variables. A *p*-level of .05 was set for all analyses.

RESULTS

Due to missing data and univariate outliers, a total of 219 students (118 boys and 101 girls) were included in the final sample. Table 1 shows the descriptive statistics. In general, the students reported moderate levels of self-efficacy (*Mean* = 4.00), enjoyment (*Mean* = 3.22), and rating of perceived exertion (*Mean* = 13.53).

Relationships among Children's Self-efficacy, Enjoyment, and Ratings of Perceived Exertion

Table 2 demonstrates the results of simple correlations among children's self-efficacy, enjoyment, and ratings of perceived exertion. The results revealed that self-efficacy, enjoyment, and ratings of perceived exertion were positively related to one another (self-efficacy and enjoyment, $r = 0.45$; self-efficacy and ratings of perceived exertion, $r = 0.21$; enjoyment and ratings of perceived exertion, $r = 0.14$; all $p < 0.05$).

Table 1. Descriptive Statistics by Grade and Gender (N = 219)

	Grade	Gender	Mean	Standard Deviation	Number
Self-efficacy	3	Girls	3.87	0.73	37
		Boys	3.92	0.80	51
		Total	3.90	0.77	88
	4	Girls	4.04	0.82	39
		Boys	4.12	0.55	40
		Total	4.08	0.69	79
	5	Girls	4.13	0.74	25
		Boys	3.99	0.93	27
		Total	4.06	0.84	52
	Total	Girls	4.00	0.77	101
		Boys	4.00	0.76	18
		Total	4.00	0.76	219
Enjoyment	3	Girls	3.24	0.64	37
		Boys	3.25	0.74	51
		Total	3.25	0.70	88
	4	Girls	3.11	0.82	39
		Boys	3.26	0.69	40
		Total	3.18	0.76	79
	5	Girls	3.13	0.84	25
		Boys	3.36	0.67	27
		Total	3.25	0.76	52
	Total	Girls	3.16	0.76	101
		Boys	3.28	0.71	118
		Total	3.22	0.73	219
Rating of Perceived Exertion	3	Girls	14.08	4.15	37
		Boys	13.76	3.70	51
		Total	13.90[b]	3.87	88
	4	Girls	14.67	3.07	39
		Boys	13.45	3.71	40
		Total	14.05[b]	3.45	79
	5	Girls	12.56	3.58	25
		Boys	12.00	2.77	27
		Total	12.27[a]	3.17	52
	Total	Girls	13.93	3.68	101
		Boys	13.25	3.56	118
		Total	13.57	3.62	219

Notes. [a, b]: there is a significant difference between the groups, $p < .01$.

Regression analysis further yielded that self-efficacy was a significant positive predictor for ratings of perceived exertion ($ß = 0.21$, $t = 3.093$,

$p < 0.01$). However, enjoyment did not emerge as a predictor of ratings of perceived exertion ($\beta = 0.05$, $t = 0.72$, $p > 0.05$).

Table 2. Correlation among Children's Self-efficacy, Enjoyment, and RPE

	Mean	Standard Deviation	1	2	3
1. Self-efficacy	4.00	.76	-	$.21^{**}$	$.14^{*}$
2. Enjoyment	3.22	.73	-	-	$.45^{**}$
3. RPE	13.57	3.621	-	-	-

Notes. $^{*}p < .05$; $^{**}p < .01$.

Gender and Grade Differences

The two-way multivariate analysis of variance yielded a significant main effect for grade, F (2, 213) = 4.56, $p < 0.01$. Follow-up univariate tests indicated that third (*Mean* = 13.92) and fourth (*Mean* = 14.05) grade children reported significantly higher ratings of perceived exertion than fifth (*Mean* = 12.28) grade children while playing exergames. However, the multivariate analysis of variance did not reveal a main effect for sex.

DISCUSSION

Regular physical activity participation has been associated with decreased prevalence of overweight, improved health-related physical fitness, and improved mental health. The present study attempted to investigate the relationships of children's self-efficacy, enjoyment, and ratings of perceived exertion during an exergaming program. It also examined grade and gender differences in these outcome variables among elementary school children.

Descriptive data revealed children reported moderate levels of self-efficacy, enjoyment, and ratings of perceived exertion which indicates that children in this study liked playing exergames and actively participated in the exergaming activities. These findings support literature indicating exergaming is beneficial for children and that playing exergames can bring children pleasant and enjoyable experiences (Gao et al., 2011).

Correlation analyses revealed significant positive relationships among all the study variables. Specifically, self-efficacy, enjoyment, and ratings of perceived exertion were positively related to one another, and therefore the results supported the first research hypothesis. The results imply that children who were competent playing exergames were more likely to enjoy the gameplay and put forth more effort. This finding echoes previous studies examining the relationships between exergaming and motivational factors (Gao et al., 2012; Gao et al., 2013).

Not surprisingly, self-efficacy was a significant positive predictor for ratings of perceived exertion, while enjoyment failed to predict ratings of perceived exertion. Specifically, those who felt more competent were also more likely to exert more effort when playing exergaming. The finding is in line with the extant studies indicating self-efficacy to be a correlate for children's physical activity levels (Boyce & Bingham, 1997; Dishman et al., 2004; Gao et al., 2008). Based on Bandura's definition of self-efficacy (Bandura, 1997), teachers could enhance children's self-efficacy in exergaming through a range of practices. First, teachers shall clarify the teaching objectives and structure of the course content for the children at the beginning of teaching, so children can set appropriate learning goals. For example, Mainwaring and Krasnow (2010) indicated that clear class goals and structure prompted self-efficacy in teaching dance. Thus, transparent teaching may contribute to children's self-efficacy. Second, teachers may encourage children and provide them with positive feedback. Research shows that feedback and self-efficacy are related (Saemi, Porter, Ghotbi-Varzaneh, Zarghami, & Maleki, 2012). Positive feedback and encouragement can build up children's confidence and let them believe that they are competent playing exergames. Finally, teachers can guide children in setting realistic learning goals for themselves. Unrealistic learning goals are not beneficial to the development of individuals' self-efficacy (Pajares, 1996). Therefore, it is necessary for teachers to assist their students to find easy goals when beginning a novel task. Within an exergaming curriculum, teachers can help children set easier goals at the beginning of the intervention, which aid in enhancing self-efficacy.

The finding that enjoyment failed to emerge as a predictor of ratings of perceived exertion was unexpected, as enjoyment has been linked to physical activity participation among young adults in previous studies (Epstein et al., 2007; Dishman et al., 2005). Given the fact that the relationship between enjoyment and perceived effort during exergaming remains largely unexplored, this study contributed to the literature stating that individuals' perceptions of enjoyment might not relate to the perceived effort. It may be that a high level of perceived enjoyment is not necessarily associated with high effort during a workout. We recommend that this factor be explored further among different populations in the future.

Additionally, fifth grade children reported significantly lower ratings of perceived exertion than third and fourth grade children. That is, children in lower grades tended to report exerting more effort than children in higher grades (i.e., fifth grade students). It is possible that older children had more exergaming experience than younger children and, thus, less effort was demanded during exergame gameplay. Another plausible explanation for this result might relate to different motor development levels of the children. In general, older children are more physically developed than the younger ones. The lower motor development level of younger children might provide extra challenges for the third and fourth grade students to perform in exergaming as compared to the fifth grade children. This difference may cause varied levels of perceived effort during performance of the same activity. More research is needed in the future to examine this speculation.

No significant gender differences were seen in the present study. One possible reason for this finding may be related to the special design of exergaming. For example, exergaming is designed to provide options for all abilities and competences to play (Molina, 2004).

Regardless of the gender of the children, exergaming creates an environment of physical activities that can benefit everybody. This characteristic may explain why both boys and girls equally enjoyed the exergaming and had similar perceived energy expenditure and self-efficacy in this study. More studies are warranted, however, because of the inconsistent findings on gender differences among the exergaming literature (Duncan & Dick, 2012; Siegel, Haddock, Dubois, & Wilkin, 2009).

Finally, future research should recruit a large number of diverse children from different schools to increase the accuracy and generalizability of the findings. These studies should look to include other psychosocial variables, such as social support and achievement goals to increase our knowledge regarding how to enhance the learning experiences for school children during exergame play.

Conclusion

Findings from the present study suggest that elementary school children who were confident playing exergames enjoyed the activities and were likely to provide more effort in their participation; theoretically increasing energy expenditure. Children's self-efficacy appeared to be an important factor predicting their physical activity levels and should be emphasized when promoting exergaming during physical education. However, enjoyment might also be slightly related to elementary school children's ratings of perceived exertion during exergaming. Further study is warranted for finding the specific variance contribution of enjoyment through assessment of ethnically diverse children from different schools. In addition, the future research should examine the motor development level of the children when investigating their psychosocial correlates to the participation of exergaming for a better understanding of age differences.

References

American Heart Association. (2011). *American heart association recommendations for physical activity in adults.* Retrieved from: http://www.heart.org/HEARTORG/GettingHealthy/PhysicalActivity/StartWalking/American-Heart-Association-Recommendations-for-Physical-Activity-in-Adults_UCM_307976_Article.jsp. Published June 9, 2011.

Bailey, B., & McInnis, K. (2011). Energy cost of exergaming: A comparison of the energy cost of 6 forms of exergaming. *Archives of Pediatrics and Adolescent Medicine, 165*(7), 597-602.

Bandura A. (1997). *Self-efficacy: The exercise of control.* New York, NY: Worth Publishers.

Borg, G. (1973). Perceived exertion: A note on history and methods. *Medicine & Science in Sports & Exercise*, *5*(2), 90-93.

Bosch, P., Poloni, J., Thornton, A., & Lynskey, J. (2012). The heart rate response to Nintendo Wii boxing in young adults. *Cardiopulmonary Physical Therapy Journal, 23*(2), 13-18.

Boyce, B., & Bingham, S. (1997). The effects of self-efficacy and goal setting on bowling performance. *Journal of Teaching in Physical Education, 16*(3), 312-323.

Chen, M., Fan, X., & Moe, S. (2002). Criterion-related validity of the Borg ratings of perceived exertion scale in healthy individuals: a meta-analysis. *Journal of Sports Sciences, 20*(11), 873-889.

Coulter, M., & Woods, C. (2011). An exploration of children's perceptions and enjoyment of school-based physical activity and physical education. *Journal of Physical Activity and Health, 8*(5), 645-654.

Couture, R., Jerome, W., & Tihanyi, J. (1999). Can associative and dissociative strategies affect the swimming performance of recreational swimmers? *The Sport Psychologist, 13*(3), 334.

Devereaux, J., Pack, M, Piccott, V., Whitten, K., Basset, F., & Rohr L. (2012). Comparison of rates of perceived exertion between active video games and traditional exercise. *International Journal of Sports Medicine, 13*(3), 133-140.

Dishman, R. (1994). Prescribing exercise intensity for healthy adults using perceived exertion. *Medicine & Science in Sport & Exercise, 26*(9), 1087-1094.

Dishman, R., Motl, R., Sauders, R., Felton, G., Ward, D.S., Dowda, M., & Pate, R. (2004). Self-efficacy partially mediates the effect of a school-based physical-activity intervention among adolescent girls. *Preventive Medicine, 38*(5), 628-636.

Dishman, R., Motl, R., Sauders, R., Felton, G., Ward, D.S., Dowda, M., & Pate, R. (2005). Enjoyment mediates effects of a school-based physical-activity intervention. *Medicine & Science in Sport & Exercise, 37*(3), 478-487.

Donnelly, J.E., Jacobsen, D.J., Whatley, J.E., Hill, J.O., Swift, L.L., Cherrington, A.,…Reed, G. (1996). Nutrition and physical activity program to attenuate obesity and promote physical and metabolic fitness in elementary school children. *Obesity Research, 4*(3), 229-243.

Duncan, M., & Dick, S. (2012). Energy expenditure and enjoyment of exergaming: A comparison of the Nintendo Wii and the gamercize power stepper in young adults. *Medicina Sportiva, 16*(3), 92-98.

Epstein, L., Paluch, R., Roemmich, J., & Beecher M. (2007). Family-based obesity treatment, then and now: Twenty-five years of pediatric obesity treatment. *Health Psychology, 26*(4), 381-391.

Fitzsimmons, P., Landers, D., Thomas, J., & van der Mars, H. (1991). Does self-efficacy predict performance in experienced weightlifters? *Research Quarterly for Exercise and Sport, 62*(4), 424-431.

Fogel, V., Miltenberger, R., Graves, R., & Koehler, S. (2010). The effects of exergaming on physical activity among inactive children in a physical education classroom. *Journal of Applied Behavior Analysis, 43*(4), 591-600.

Gao, Z., & Chen, S. (2014). Are field-based exergames useful in preventing childhood obesity? A systematic review. *Obesity Reviews, 15,* 676-691. doi: 10.1111/obr.12164.

Gao, Z., Hannon, J., Newton, M., & Huang, C. (2011). Effects of curricular activity on students' situational motivation and physical activity levels. *Research Quarterly for Exercise and Sport, 82*(3), 536-544.

Gao, Z., Huang, C., Liu, T., & Xiong, W. (2012). Impact of interactive dance games on urban children's physical activity correlates and behavior. *Journal of Exercise Science & Fitness, 10*(2), 107-115.

Gao, Z., Lochbaum, M., & Podlog L. (2011). Self-efficacy as a mediator of children's achievement motivation and in-class physical activity. *Perceptual & Motor Skills, 113*(3), 969-981.

Gao, Z., Newton, M., & Carson, R. (2008). Students' motivation, physical activity levels, & health-related physical fitness in middle school physical education. *Middle Grades Research Journal, 3*(4), 21-39.

Gao, Z., Podlog, L., & Huang, C. (2013). Associations among children's situational motivation, physical activity participation, and enjoyment in an interactive dance game. *Journal of Sport and Health Science, 2,* 122-128.

Gao, Z., Zhang, T., & Stodden, D. (2013). Children's physical activity levels and psychological correlated in interactive dance versus aerobic dance. *Journal of Sport and Health Science, 2,* 146-151.

Graves, L., Ridgers, N., Williams, K., Stratton, G., Atkinson, G., & Cable, N. (2010). The physiological cost and enjoyment of Wii Fit in adolescents, young adults, and older adults. *Journal of Physical Activity and Health, 7*(3), 393-401.

Impellizzeri, F., Rampinini, E., & Marcora, S. Physiological assessment of aerobic training in soccer. *Journal of Sports Sciences, 23*(6), 583-592.

Lanningham-Foster, L., Foster, R., McCrady, S., Jensen, T., Mitre, N., & Levine, J. (2009). Activity-promoting video games and increased energy expenditure. *Journal of Pediatrics, 154*(6), 819-823.

Liang, H., Motl, R., McAuley, E., & Konopack, J. (2007). Effects of self-efficacy on physical activity enjoyment in college-aged women. *International Journal of Behavioral Medicine, 14*(2), 92-96.

Mainwaring, L., & Krasnow, D. (2010). Teaching the dance class: strategies to enhance skill acquisition, mastery and positive self-image. *Journal of Dance Education, 10*(1), 14-21.

Malherbe, D., Steel, H., & Theron, W. (2003). The contribution of self-efficacy and outcome expectations in the prediction of exercise adherence. *South African Journal for Research in Sport, Physical Education, and Recreation, 25*(1), 71-82.

McAuley, E. (1985). Success and Causality in Sport: The Influence of Perception. *Journal of Sport Psychology, 7*(1), 13-22.

Molina, A. (2004). A "fitness" revolution? *American Fitness, 22*(2), 26-27.

Motl, R.W., Dishman, R.K., Ward, D.S., Saunders, R.P., Dowda, M., Felton, G., & Pate, R.R. (2002). Examining social-cognitive determinants of intention and physical activity among Black and White adolescent girls using structural equation modeling. *Health Psychology, 21*(5), 459-467.

Mullins, N., Tessmer, K., Mccarroll, M., & Peppel, B. (2012). Physiological and perceptual responses to Nintendo® Wii Fit™ in young and older adults. *International Journal of Exercise Science, 5*(1), 79-92.

National Association of Sport and Physical Education. (2009). *Moving into the future: National standards for physical education* (2nd ed.). Reston, VA: Human Kinetics.

National Institutes of Health. (2010). How much physical activity should your family get? Retrieved from: http://www.nhlbi.nih.gov/health/public/heart/obesity/wecan/get-active/physical-activity-guidelines.htm.

Ning, W., Gao, Z., & Lodewyk, K. (2012). Associations between socio-motivational factors, physical education activity levels and physical activity behavior among youth. *International Council for Health, Physical Education, Recreation, Sport, and Dance - Journal of Research, 7*(2), 3-10.

O'Loughlin, E., Dugas, E., Sabiston, C., & O'Loughlin, J. (2012). Prevalence and correlates of exergaming in youth. *Pediatrics, 130*(5), 806-814.

Ommundsen, Y., Page, A., Ku, P., & Cooper, A. (2008). Cross-cultural, age and gender validation of a computerized questionnaire measuring personal, social and environmental associations with children's physical activity: The European Youth Heart Study. *International Journal of Behavioral Nutrition and Physical Activity, 5,* 29.

Pajares, F. (1996). Self-efficacy beliefs in academic settings. *Review of Education Research, 66*(4), 543-78.

Pollock, B.S., Barkley, J.E., Potenzini, N., De Salvo, R.M., Buser, S.L., Otterstetter, R., & Juvancic-Heltzel, J.A. (2012). Validity of Borg ratings of perceived exertion during active video game play. *International Journal of Exercise Science, 5*(4), 164-170.

Saemi, E., Porter, J., Ghotbi-Varzaneh, A., Zarghami, M., & Maleki, F. (2012). Knowledge of results after relatively good trials enhances self-efficacy and motor learning. *Psychology of Sport and Exercise, 13*(4), 378-382.

Sallis, J., Prochaska, J., & Taylor, W. (2000). A review of correlates of physical activity of children and adolescents. *Medicine & Science in Sport & Exercise, 32*(5), 963-975.

Siegel, S., Haddock, B., Dubois, A., & Wilkin, L. (2009). Active video/arcade games (Exergaming) and energy expenditure in college students. *International Journal of Exercise Science, 2*(3), 165-174.

Skatrud-Mickelson, M., Benson, J., Hannon, J., & Askew, E. (2011). A comparison of subjective and objective measures of physical exertion. *Journal of Sports Sciences, 29*(15), 1635-1644.

US Department of Health and Human Services (USDHHS). (2006). Health, United States, 2006: With Chartbook on Trends in the Health of Americans. Retrieved from: MEDLINE.

Vandewater, E., Rideout, V., Wartella, E., Huang, X., Lee, J., & Shim, M. (2007). Digital childhood: Electronic media and technology use among infants, toddlers, and preschoolers. *Pediatrics, 119*(5), e1006-15.

Vuillerme, N., & Hintzy, F. (2007). Effects of a 200 W-15 min cycling exercise on postural control during quiet standing in healthy young adults. *European Journal of Applied Physiology, 100*(2), 169-175.

Wergel-Kolmert, U., & Wohlfart, B. (1999). Day-to-day variation in oxygen consumption and energy expenditure during submaximal treadmill walking in female adolescents. *Clinical Physiology (Oxford, England), 19*(2), 161-168.

In: Physical Activity Behaviors … ISBN: 978-1-63483-635-7
Editors: Zan Gao and Zachary Pope

Chapter 6

HIGH SCHOOL STUDENTS' SITUATIONAL INTEREST AND PHYSICAL ACTIVITY LEVELS IN EXERGAMING

Cédric Roure[1], Denis Pasco[2], Zachary Pope[3] and Zan Gao[3]

[1]Catholic University of Louvain-la-Neuve, Louvain-la-Neuve, Belgium
[2]European University of Brittany, Brest, France
[3]University of Minnesota-Twin Cities, Minneapolis, MN, US

ABSTRACT

The benefits and challenges of integrating exergames in schools to promote young children's physical activity and interest have been evident. Yet, such investigations remain unexplored among older adolescents. Thus, the purpose of this study was to examine the relationships between high school students' situational interest and physical activity levels during exergame play, as well as investigate the gender and grade differences on the study variables. A total of 60 (32 girls; Mean = 16.17 years, *SD* = 1.17) 10th through 12th grade students participated in one session of Reflex Ridge, part of the Xbox 360 *Kinect Adventures* game. Students' physical activity levels were measured by Actigraph accelerometers with percentages of time spent in sedentary, light physical activity and moderate-to-vigorous physical activity as the outcome variables. They also responded to the validated Situational Interest Scale (measuring novelty, challenge, attention demand, exploration intention, and instant enjoyment) at the end of the session. Regression and path analysis indicated that attention demand was a significant positive predictor for moderate-to-vigorous physical activity (ß = 0.41, $p < 0.05$ accounting for 16.7% of the variance) while novelty was a marginally significant positive predictor for light physical activity (ß = 0.25, $p < 0.06$ accounting for 13.4% of the variance). Multivariate analysis of variance revealed no gender effect on sedentary, light physical activity and moderate-to-vigorous physical activity, and that 11th grade students spent significantly higher percentages of time in moderate-to-vigorous physical activity than 10th and 12th grade students (F (6,104) = 2.51, $p < 0.05$). Findings suggested high school students displayed higher moderate-to-vigorous physical activity when they felt the activity demanded greater attention but demonstrated higher light physical activity when they deemed the activity only provided novelty. The motivational power of exergaming may be an opportunity to intervene and attenuate the increasingly sedentary daily activities currently engaged in by adolescents. However, physical educators should consider the motivational power of attention (i.e., cognitive) demand to physically engage high school students in exergaming experiences.

Keywords: situational interest, attention demand, exploration intention, instant enjoyment

INTRODUCTION

Playing video games is commonplace among children and adolescents daily routine. According to a large-scale study with a nationally representative sample, 88% of American youth between ages 8 to 18 years play video games at least occasionally (Gentile, 2009). Further, research has indicated playing sedentary video games have long been associated with various risks for both mental and physical health including (1) provocation of seizures, tendon injuries, and social introversion related to game addiction (Fischer, 1994; Dorman, 1997); (2) hostility, aggressive behaviors, effects on school performance related to playing violent video games (Gentile, Lynch, Linder, & Walsh, 2004); and (3) increased body mass index related to overplaying sedentary video games (Vandewater, Shim, & Caplovitz, 2004).

A decade ago, a new type of video game genre called 'exergames' or 'active video games' emerged. Exergames refer to video games that are also a form of exercise (Gao & Chen, 2014). Exergames necessitate physical activity as a means of interacting with the game. In the last decade, researchers have extensively investigated the potential of exergames to promote children/adolescents' physical activity participation. In a recent meta-analysis on the effects of exergames on children/adolescents' physiological and psychological health-related outcomes, Gao, Chen, Pasco, and Pope (2015) indicated that exergames (1) have a large effect on children/adolescents' physiological and psychological outcomes as compared to sedentary behaviors; (2) produce the equivalent magnitude of effect as light-to-moderate-intensity physical activity; and (3) are more attractive and enjoyable for children/adolescents in comparison with traditional physical activity. Taken together, these findings suggest that exergames are a viable option to promote children/adolescents' physical activity and health based on their attractiveness in comparison with traditional physical activity.

Despite the attractiveness of exergames among youth, few studies investigated children/adolescents' experiences of exergaming through the lens of the situational interest (Sun, 2012; Sun, 2013; Huang & Gao, 2013). Situational interest has been defined as an activity's appealing effect on an individual(s) (Hidi & Anderson, 1992) and emerges from an instant person-activity interaction in which the person recognizes a specific feature of this activity while being engaged in it (Mitchell, 1993). According to Hidi and Harackiewicz (2000), a highly interesting activity can immediately attract individuals' attention and provide positive feelings about the activity. Within the context of physical activity, Chen, Darst and Pangrazi (1999, 2001) identified five sources of situational interest: novelty, challenge, attention demand, exploration intention, and instant enjoyment.

Novelty is conceptualized as a gap between information known and unknown in an activity (i.e., information deficiency). According to Spielberger and Starr (1994), novelty functions to elicit individuals' participation in this activity. Challenge has been defined as the level of difficulty relative to one's own ability and has been identified as a motivational factor that may predispose student's engagement in an activity (Harter, 1978). Regarding attention demand and exploration intention, these constructs represent the stimulation generated by the person-activity interaction that create a perception of situational interest in the activity. According to Deci (1992), the power of the preceding two constructs increases the individual's intrinsic motivation to engage in the activity. Finally, instant enjoyment refers to individuals' emotional engagement with an activity (Hedi & Anderson, 1992).

Sun (2012) explored the impact of an exergaming unit on students' physical activity levels and situational interest compared to a traditional fitness-education unit in elementary school physical education. Fourth grade students participated in a four-week exergaming unit and a four-week fitness unit. Results showed that the children's physical activity levels during the exergaming unit was significantly lower than in the fitness unit but did indicate students' situational interest during exergaming to be significantly higher than in the fitness unit at the beginning and end of the intervention. Sun (2013) conducted a follow-up study with the same group. Fifth grade students from the previous study below participated in an exergaming unit. The results indicated that students' physical activity intensity increased over time while their situational interest decreased significantly with the exception of attention demand and instant enjoyment. Finally, Huang and Gao (2013) found that novelty was a significant predictor of moderate-to-vigorous physical activity during exergame play with a population of 135 middle school students ranging from 12 to 15 years old. Students participated in an exergaming unit (Dance Dance Revolution) for two weeks. Results suggested that students demonstrate higher physical activity levels if they feel the exergames provided new information (i.e., novelty).

Given the preceding literature review and available evidence, it is clear exergames have great potential to promote children's physical activity participation and situational interest in physical education. Yet, such investigations remain unexplored among older adolescents. Thus, the purpose of this study was to examine the relationships between high school students' situational interest and physical activity levels during exergame play, as well as investigate the gender and grade differences for the study variables.

METHODS

Participants

A cross-sectional design was used to examine the relationships between objectively-measured physical activity levels and self-report situational interest in exergaming. The study was conducted in an inner city high school in a medium-sized metropolitan area of the northwest region of France. Participants were 10th to 12th grade students' ages 15-20 years (N = 60; 28 boys, 32 girls; $Mean_{age}$ = 16.17, SD = 1.17). They participated in one session of Reflex Ridge, part of the Xbox 360 *Kinect Adventures* game. Following the University Institutional Review Board and school district requirements, student assent forms and parental consent were obtained. All participants were eligible to participate in the study, as the game has limited physical risks. Therefore, all of the students participated in the study.

Instruments

Physical Activity Levels. To collect student physical activity levels, the researchers utilized Actigraph GT3X+ accelerometers (Pensacola, FL, USA). The Actigraph GT3X+ measures motion in three dimensions and provides triaxial vector data in metabolic equivalents. It is 4.6 x 3.3 x 1.5 cm in size and can be worn on the wrist, waist (hip), arm or ankle. In this study, students wore the accelerometer on the hip using an elastic belt. Data from the hip has been shown to be the best location for providing data to detect a range of everyday activities (Cleland et al., 2013). The GT3X+ is widely used in physical activity research and has demonstrated acceptable criterion validity and reliability for recording physical activity in the field and converting activity counts into different intensity levels of physical activity (Flynn, Coe, Larsen, Rider, Conger, & Bassett, 2014). Accelerations from the Actigraph GT3X+ were converted into activity counts, summed and recorded using a specified interval of time called an 'epoch' ranging from 5 seconds to 1 minute. In the present study, the epoch was set at 5 seconds. Cut points were established using Puyau, Adolph, Vohra, and Butte (2002) study to determine sedentary (0-399 counts per 30s), light (400-1599 counts per 30s), and moderate-to-vigorous physical activity (≥1600 counts per 30s). Students' percentage of time spent in moderate-to-vigorous physical activity, light physical activity and sedentary were used as the outcome variables.

Situational Interest. The French 19-item Situational Interest Scale (Roure, Pasco, & Kermarrec, in press) was used to measure students' situational interest during the exergaming session. The scale includes five situational interest constructs: Novelty (i.e., what the researchers did today was new to me), Instant Enjoyment (i.e., what the researchers did was enjoyable for me), Exploration Intention (i.e., I wanted to analyze and have a better handle on what the researchers were learning today), Attention demand (i.e., what the researchers were learning demanded my high attention), and Challenge (i.e., what the researchers were learning was hard for me to do). The items are randomly arranged and each is attached to a five-point Likert scale ranging from 1 = *strongly disagree* to 5 = *strongly agree*. Roure et al., (2013) established the construct validity of the French Situational Interest Scale using exploratory and confirmatory factor analyses. They also reported internal consistency (Cronbach's alpha) for novelty (0.83), instant enjoyment (0.84), exploration intention (0.79), attention demand (0.76), challenge (0.77), and total interest (0.85) among middle and high school students.

Procedures

The data were collected at the end of the 2014 school year, the researchers did not have a chance to implement the exergaming session into physical education class curriculum. Instead, the exergaming program was setup in a large empty room beside the school library. Students were informed about the opportunity to participate in the study through paper information and flyers. If the students expressed interest to participate, they were required to enroll in the program through the librarian. Then, the researchers created a schedule with two students playing for a 30-minute exergaming session. Data were collected during one week. Before the students engaged in exergame play, the researchers collected their demographic information such as grade, age, gender, height and weight. Such information was needed to initiate accelerometers in order to collect accurate physical activity measures and, as such, was entered into the ActiLife software prior to placing the accelerometers on the adolescents. After placing the accelerometers to the students, the researchers introduced and demonstrated how to play the exergame. Students played the Reflex Ridge game one time with two players in the spilt screen. Reflex Ridge is one of the top ten Kinect games. It is a track-and-field inspired game played on a moving platform in an environment similar to a wooden roller coaster or mine cart. Players raced on a platform, jumped over hurdles, leaned away from obstacles, and limboed to avoid hitting their heads on low beams. Jumping in place made the platform move faster along its rail. Adventure pins were earned by avoiding obstacles or touching ones scattered throughout the course. The game was timed, with extra time left over at the end of the course added to the Adventure pin total. In the present study, the students competed one to another to collect more pins. In addition, the students reported their situational interest at the end of the session.

Data Analyses

Students' responses to the situational interest scale were aggregated to the five constructs (novelty, instant enjoyment, exploration intention, attention demand, and challenge). Means and standard deviations were calculated for each situational interest construct, moderate-to-vigorous physical activity, light physical activity and sedentary. Then, a multivariate analysis of variance was performed to examine the effect of gender and grade on students' moderate-to-vigorous physical activity, light physical activity and sedentary, respectively. Finally, three stepwise multiple regression analyses were used to determine if any of the five situational interest dimensions predicted students' moderate-to-vigorous physical activity, light physical activity and sedentary, respectively.

RESULTS

Descriptive Statistics

Descriptive statistics for each variable are presented in Table 1. As shown in Table 1, means scores for novelty, exploration intention and attention demand were slightly above the midpoint (i.e., 10). The mean score for instant enjoyment was the highest (13.93) while the exergaming session was not a challenge for students as referenced by the lower mean score of 5.82. Additionally, students' spent more than 78% of their time in moderate to vigorous physical activity during exergame play.

Table 2 presents descriptive statistics for each variable by gender and grade. Results indicate that average percentage of time in moderate-to-vigorous physical activity during the exergaming session was 78.09% and 79.35% for girls and boys, respectively.

A multivariate analysis of variance was performed to examine the effect of gender and grade on students' moderate to vigorous physical activity. Results revealed a significant main effect for grade, $\lambda = 0.76$, $F(6,104) = 2.51$, $p = 0.02$, $n^2 = 0.12$.

Pairwise comparisons indicated significant differences between 10th and 11th graders as well as 11th and 12th graders but no difference between 10th and 12th graders. No significant gender differences were found in the percentage of time spent at different physical activity levels, however (p = 0.85 for sedentary, 0.87 for light and 0.69 moderate-to-vigorous physical activity levels respectively).

Table 1. Descriptive Statistics for Each Variable

Variable	Novelty	Instant Enjoyment	Exploration Intention	Attention Demand	Challenge	MVPA	Light PA	Sedentary PA
Mean	10.52	13.93	11.33	11.88	5.82	78.68	3.65	17.77
SD	3.61	1.69	2.73	3.19	2.16	6.08	3.95	6.43

Note. SD = Standard deviation; MVPA = students' percentage of time spent in moderate to vigorous physical activity.

Table 2. Descriptive Statistics for Each Variable by Gender and Grade

Variable	Gender		Grade		
	Boys (n = 28)	Girls (n = 32)	10 (n = 30)	11 (n = 22)	12 (n = 8)
	M (SD)	*M (SD)*	*M (SD)*	*M (SD)*	*M (SD)*
Novelty	10.36 (3.46)	10.66 (3.79)	10.60 (3.51)	10.05 (3.55)	11.50 (4.37)
Instant Enjoyment	14.00 (1.46)	13.88 (1.89)	13.70 (1.95)	14.32 (0.78)	13.75 (2.43)
Exploration Intention	11.93 (2.73)	10.81 (2.67)	11.37 (2.76)	12.00 (2.11)	9.37* (3.50)
Attention Demand	13.04 (3.00)	10.87 (3.05)	11.37 (3.48)	12.55 (2.66)	12.00 (3.46)
Challenge	5.86 (2.12)	5.78 (2.24)	6.10 (2.25)	5.50 (1.82)	5.63 (2.82)
MVPA	79.35 (6.22)	78.09 (5.98)	77.26 (5.18)	81.91* (6.07)	75.12 (5.79)
Light PA	3.18 (0.80)	3.38 (0.91)	4.72 (0.75)	2.23 (0.84)	2.90 (1.43)
Sedentary PA	18.55 (1.31)	18.93 (1.50)	17.85 (1.23)	15.98 (1.38)	22.40 (2.33)

Note. MVPA = students' percentage of time spent in moderate to vigorous physical activity; *There is a significant difference between the groups, $p < 0.05$.

Table 3. Correlations between variable

Variable	Novelty	Instant Enjoyment	Exploration Intention	Attention Demand	Challenge	MVPA	Light PA	Sedentary PA
Novelty	-	0.18	0.27*	0.26*	0.01	-0.07	0.20	-0.05
Instant Enjoyment		-	0.49**	0.48**	-0.11	-0.00	0.01	0.06
Exploration Intention			-	0.57**	0.30**	0.19	-0.08	-0.09
Attention Demand				-	0.28*	0.30*	-0.21	-0.09
Challenge					-	0.01	0.01	-0.00

Note. MVPA = students' percentage of time spent in moderate to vigorous physical activity. $^{*}p < 0.05$, $^{**}p < 0.01$.

Pairwise comparisons indicated significant differences between 12th grade students and both 10th and 11th grade students on exploration intention ($p < 0.05$). No significant differences were found for novelty, instant enjoyment, attention demand and challenge based on students' grade levels.

Correlation and Regression Analyses

Correlation analyses indicated that the five constructs of situational interest are significantly related to one another. However, attention demand was the only dimension significantly related to moderate-to-vigorous physical activity (Table 3).

A stepwise multiple regression analysis was performed to determine how students' situational interest dimensions predicted their physical activity levels. Results indicated that attention demand emerged as a significant predictor of moderate-to-vigorous physical activity, $ß = 0.41$, $p < 0.05$ accounting for 16.7% of the variance for this intensity of physical activity while novelty was found to be a marginally significant predictor of students' light physical activity, $ß = 0.25$, $p < 0.06$ accounting for 13.4% of the variance in this variable.

Discussion

Researchers have suggested that exergames may present an opportunity to promote children/adolescents' physical activity especially as an alternative to sedentary activities (Gao et al., 2015). Based on the attractiveness of exergames among children and adolescents, this study was designed to examine the impact of playing an exergame on high school students' physical activity levels and situational interest by gender and grade. Students participated in one session of Reflex Ridge, part of the Xbox 360 *Kinect Adventures* game. Students' physical activity levels were measured with Actigraph GT3X+ accelerometers with percentage of time spent in sedentary, light physical activity, and moderate-to-vigorous physical activity as the outcome variables while students self-reported their situational interest during the session using the French Situational Interest Scale (Roure et al., 2013). Data indicated that students spent 78% of the session time in moderate-to-vigorous physical activity when playing the exergame with no significant differences between boys and girls. The findings also indicated that 11th grade students spent significantly higher percentages of time in moderate-to-vigorous physical activity than 10th and 12th grade students while attention demand emerged as a predictor for moderate-to-vigorous physical activity. Finally, novelty was marginally predictive of light physical activity.

When Trost et al., (2002) reported age and gender differences in objectively measured daily physical activity among youth, they found that (1) Physical activity declines rapidly during childhood and adolescence; and (2) boys engaged in significantly greater moderate-to-vigorous physical activity participation than girls (with the exception of grades 1-3). Our study revealed that high school students' experiences during exergame play do not follow this trend. Students spent most of their time in moderate-to-vigorous physical activity when playing the exergame as 11th grade students were more active than 10th and 12th grade students in addition to boys and girls were equally active. This might be due to the attractiveness of exergaming among youth—especially in a competitive situation (i.e., side-by-side two-player action). Previous studies (Huang & Gao, 2013; Sun, 2012) provide empirical evidence to support the motivating nature of exergaming. Sun (2012) found high levels of instant enjoyment, exploration intention and challenge among elementary children when they played exergames in class. Huang and Gao (2013) reported high levels of novelty as the sole predictor for moderate-to-vigorous physical activity among middle school students. Exergaming provided a unique and new experience in which boys and girls were challenged, explored the game situations, and focused on key elements of the games that led to high levels of enjoyment. As Sun (2012) concluded: "The motivation derived from the exergaming activity can be conceived to be representative of typical intrinsic motivation rarely seen in children and even older learners" (p. 217). Therefore, the motivational power of exergaming may be an opportunity to attenuate the increase of sedentary activities throughout childhood and adolescence.

The findings also revealed that high school students' perceived attention demand was a predictor of their time spent in moderate-to-vigorous physical activity. Additionally novelty approached significance for the prediction of students' light physical activity. Huang and Gao (2013) found that novelty was the only significant predictor of students' moderate-to-vigorous physical activity suggesting that middle school students would engage in higher amounts physical activity if they felt the exergame provides new information. Our results show that, although novelty may be enough to physically engage middle school students in exergames, it is not enough for high school students. Further, according to the findings of the present study, novelty may only lead to light physical activity among this age group. In other words, high school students may not exercise at a moderate-to-vigorous physical activity level if they feel the exergame only provides novelty but not the need for increased attention demand—a fact which limits the adolescent from deriving the health benefits associated with moderate-to-vigorous physical activity. Given that exergames are not a new concept for adolescents anymore, exergames should provide attention demand to support high school students' moderate-to-vigorous physical activity.

Specifically, attention demand refers to cognitive engagement. This cognitive engagement is typically facilitated as a result of students' need to generate mental models quickly during exergame play in order to successfully navigate the game. Mental models have been defined as "a special kind of mental representation, an analog representation, which individuals generate during cognitive functioning" (Vosniadou, 1994; p. 48). According to Hayes and Silberman (2007), exergames players develop a wide range of mental models to help them decide how to succeed in various game situations. In the current study, students playing Reflex Ridge had to constantly decide which position to take on the platform and if they would have to squat or jump to avoid the obstacles or to make the platform move faster along its rail. The generation of mental models helps them to make better and faster decisions in these exergame situations. The results of this study on the role of cognitive demand are consistent with findings in previous studies (Chen & Darst, 2001). Cognitive demand is the key to physically engage high school students in exergaming experiences. Accordingly, physical educators should consider the motivational power of cognitive demand on students' physical activity levels when they use exergames.

In conclusion, the findings from this study provided evidence that exergaming can be a powerful source of situational interest motivation and lead to health benefits among high school students. However, physical educators should receive professional training to use exergames effectively to promote physical activity.

References

Chen, A., Darst, P. W., & Pangrazi, R. P. (1999). What constitutes situational interest? Validating a construct in physical education. *Measurement in Physical Education and Exercise Science, 3*, 157–180.

Chen, A., Darst, P. W., & Pangrazi, R. P. (2001). An examination of situational interest and its sources in physical education. *British Journal of Educational Psychology, 71*, 383–400.

Cleland, I., Kikhia, B., Nugent, C., Boytsov, A., Hallberg, J., Synnes, K., McClean, S., & Finlay, D. (2013). Optimal placement of accelerometers for the detection of everyday activities. *Sensors, 13*, 9183-9200.

Deci, E. L. (1992). The relation of interest to the motivation of behavior: A self-determination theory perspective. In K. A. Renninger, S. Hidi, & A. Krapp (Eds.), *The role of interest in learning and development* (pp. 43–69). Hillsdale, NJ: Lawrence Erlbaum Associates, Inc.

Dorman, S. (1997). Video and computer games: Effect on children and implications for health education. *Journal of School Health, 67*(4), 133–138.

Fisher, S. (1994). Identifying video game addiction in children and adolescents. *Addictive Behaviors, 19*(5), 545-553.

Flynn, J.L., Coe, D.P., Larsen, C.A., Rider, B.C., Conger, S.A., & Bassett, D.R Jr (2014). Detecting indoor and outdoor environments using the ActiGraph GT3X+ light sensor in children. *Medicine and Science in Sports and Exercise, 46*(1), 201-206.

Gao, Z., & Chen, S. (2014). Response to letter: No clear evidence that exergames can prevent obesity. *Obesity Reviews, 15,* 694-695.

Gao, Z., Chen, S., Pasco, D., & Pope, Z. (2015). A meta-analysis of active video games on health outcomes among children and adolescents. *Obesity reviews*. doi:10.1111/obr.12287.

Gentile, D. (2009). Pathological video-game use among youth ages 8 to 18. *Psychological Science, 20*(5), 594-602.

Gentile, D.A., Lynch, P.J., Ruh Linder, J., & Walsh, D.A. (2004). The effects of violent video game habits on adolescent hostility, aggressive behaviors, and school performance. *Journal of Adolescence, 27*(1), 5-22.

Harter, S. (1978). Pleasure derived from optimal challenge and the effects of extrinsic rewards on children's difficulty levels choices. *Child Development, 49*, 788-799.

Hayes, E., & Silberman, L. (2007). Incorporating video games into physical education. *The Journal of Physical Education, Recreation & Dance, 78*(3), 18–24.

Hidi, S., & Anderson, V. (1992). Situational interest and its impact on reading and expository writing. In K. A. Renninger, S. Hidi, & A. Krapp (Eds.), *The role of interest in learning and development* (pp. 215–238). Hillsdale, NJ: Lawrence Erlbaum Associates, Inc.

Hidi, S., & Harackiewicz, J. M. (2000). Motivating the academically unmotivated: A critical issue for the 21st century. *Review of Educational Research, 70,* 151–179.

Huang, C., & Gao, Z. (2013). Associations between students' situational interest, mastery experiences, and physical activity levels in an interactive dance game. *Psychology, Health & Medicine, 18*(2), 233-241. doi: 10.1080/13548506.2012.712703.

Puyau, M. R., Adolph, A. L., Vohra, F. A., & Butte, N. F. (2002). Validation and calibration of physical activity monitors in children. *Obesity Research, 10*, 150–157.

Roure, C, Pasco, D., & Kermarrec, G. (in press). Validation française de l'échelle mesurant l'intérêt en situation en éducation physique [French validation of the situational interest scale in physical education]. Canadian Journal of Behavioural Science.

Spielberger, C. D., & Starr, L. M. (1994). Curiosity and exploratory behavior. In H. F. O'Neil, Jr., & M. Drillings (Eds.), *Motivation: Theory and research* (pp. 221–243). Hillsdale, NJ: Lawrence Erlbaum Associates, Inc.

Sun, H. (2012). Exergaming impact on physical activity and interest in elementary school children. *Research Quarterly for Exercise and Sport, 83*(2), 212-220.

Sun, H. (2013). Impact of exergames on physical activity and motivation in elementary school students: A follow-up study. *Journal of Sport and Health Science, 2*(3), 138-145.

Trost, S. G., Pate, R. R., Sallis, J. F., Freedson, P. S., Taylor, W. C., Dowda, M., & Sirard, J. (2002). Age and gender differences in objectively measured physical activity in youth. *Medicine & Science in Sports & Exercise, 34*(2), 350-355.

Vandewater, E., Shim, M., & Caplovitz, A.G. (2004). Linking obesity and activity level with children's television and video game use. *Journal of Adolescence, 27*(1), 71-85.

Vosniadou, S. (1994). Capturing and modeling the process of conceptual change. *Learning and Instruction, 4*(1), 45–69.

In: Physical Activity Behaviors … ISBN: 978-1-63483-635-7
Editors: Zan Gao and Zachary Pope

Chapter 7

MEDIATING ROLE OF PERCEIVED COMPETENCE ON CHILDREN'S PERCEIVED EXERGAMING SKILLS, PHYSICAL ACTIVITY AND FITNESS

Jung Eun Lee[1], David F. Stodden[2], Tao Zhang[3], Alice Fang Yan[4] and Zan Gao[1]

[1]University of Minnesota-Twin Cities, Minneapolis, MN, US
[2]Department of Physical Education & Athletic Training, University of South Carolina, Columbia, SC, US
[3]University of North Texas, Denton, TX, US
[4]University of Wisconsin-Milwaukee, Milwaukee WI, US

ABSTRACT

Although an increasing number of studies have investigated the relationships among children's motor skills, perceived competence, physical activity participation and fitness in physical activity, such associations in exergaming settings remain unanswered. This study was designed to test the mediating role of perceived competence on the relations between children's perceived exergaming skills and physical activity during exergaming, as well as examine the relations between physical activity and health-related physical fitness. Participants were 236 third through fifth graders enrolled in a suburban elementary school. They participated in a 50-minute exergaming class (e.g., Wii Just Dance,

Dance Dance Revolution) per week for a semester. Participants responded to a battery of standardized questionnaires measuring their perceived exergaming skills and situational specific perceived competence at the end of one exergaming class. Children's physical activity levels were assessed by NL-1000 pedometers in three consecutive exergaming classes. Health-related physical fitness was assessed using FITNESSGRAM® tests for PACER, curl-ups, and push-ups.The results from the Structure Equation Modeling demonstrated an acceptable model fit to the data (χ^2/d.f. = 1.218, CFI = .995, RMSEA = .025). The overall variance in perceived competence, physical activity and fitness explained by the model was 8%, 11% and 3%, respectively. Perceived competence had a significant direct effect on physical activity after controlling for the effect of perceived exergaming skills. Perceived exergaming skills failed to exert direct effect on physical activity. However, the indirect effect of perceived exergaming skills on physical activity via perceived competence was small yet significant. Physical activity also had a positive direct effect on fitness. The results supported the mediating role of perceived competence on the relationship between perceived exergaming skills and physical activity in exergaming. The study implications are provided for educators and practitioners.

Keywords: Dance Dance Revolution, health-related physical fitness, moderate-to-vigorous physical activity, pedometer

INTRODUCTION

Physical inactivity is an important contributor to the childhood obesity epidemic (World Health Organization [WHO], 2013). To promote children's physical activity participation and reduce sedentary time, health professionals are utilizing innovative physical activity interventions that capitalize on children's interest in technology (Maloney, Stempel, Wood, Patraitis, & Beaudoin, 2012; Miller, Vaux-Bjerke, McDonnell, & DiPietro, 2013). Exergaming, video games that involve physical exertion and are thought of as a form of exercise, has recently been incorporated as an effective physical activity intervention in promoting children's physical activity due to its fun and engaging platform (Peng, Crouse, & Lin, 2013). Exergaming studies have demonstrated positive effects on children's physical activity and fitness (Gao, 2013; Gao, Hannan, Xiang, Stodden, & Valdez, 2013; Gao, Huang, Liu, & Xiong, 2012; Maloney et al., 2012, Peng et al., 2013). Exergaming interventions also have shown positive outcomes on children's motor skills

(Becker, 2007; Calvert, 2005; Gunter, 2005) and situational specific perceived competence (Gao et al., 2012). However, few studies have explored the complex underlying factors contributing to increased physical activity participation through exergaming based on their exergaming skill and perceived competence (Gao et al., 2012).

The development of motor skill competence has been positively associated with physical activity and health-related physical fitness (Barnett, van Beurden, Morgan, Brooks, & Beard, 2009; Lubans, Morgan, Cliff, Barnett, & Okely, 2010). Situational specific perceived competence (i.e., self-efficacy) refers to children's self-evaluative judgments about their ability to perform a certain task or learn a certain behavior. Barnett et al., (2009) demonstrated that children's motor skills and perceived competence have mutual effects on their physical activity and fitness. Additionally, Vedul-Kjelsås, Sigmundsson, Stensdotter, and Haga (2012) found that both physical fitness and motor skill significantly correlated with perceived athletic competence, and reported gender difference in this relationship as well (Vedul-Kjelsås et al., 2012). However, no known studies have addressed the relationships among these variables in an exergaming setting.

According to Competence Motivation Theory, a child's behavior can be predicted by the child's mastery competence (i.e., actual motor skills) and how a child perceives his/her skills (Harter, 1978). If a child's motor skills reach mastery level, he or she will experience increased perceived competence on those specific motor skills. Increased perceived competence will promote increased physical activity participation, which ultimately enhances skills related to physical activity behavior (Harter, 1978). In essence, motor skills need to be acquired through practice because the skills are not developed naturally (Stodden, Goodway, & Langendorfer, 2008). Consequently, exposure to physical activity will provide increased chance for skills to be developed (Fisher et al., 2005), which in turn will result in increased physical activity. Such dynamic relationships may strengthen as children across childhood and into adolescence (Stodden et al., 2008). In essence, the lack of development in skill within different physical activity domains may lead to either positive or negative trajectories of perceived competence and physical activity across time (Stodden et al., 2008). This notion applies in exergaming setting as well because exergaming is a form of physical activity, and it is likely that children with higher perceived competence in exergaming will be more physically active than children with low perceived competence.

The main purpose of this study was to examine the potential mediating effect of situational specific perceived competence on children's perceived exergaming skill and their physical activity and health-related physical fitness. Specifically, we hypothesized there would be positive associations between perceived exergaming skills, perceived competence and physical activity. We also hypothesized perceived competence would mediate the relations between perceived exergaming skills and physical activity. Lastly, we hypothesized children's physical activity would positively predict their physical fitness.

METHODS

Participants

The Participants were 344 (195 boys) 3rd, 4th and 5th grade elementary children in a suburban school in Texas. There were 121 3rd, 117 4th, and 106 5th graders ($Mean_{age}$ = 10.8, SD = 1.82, age range = 9-12; 195 boys, 149 girls). The majority of children (58%) were non-Hispanic White. Children participated in the exergaming program as a class unit with each child playing individually on a variety of exergames (e.g., Wii Sports, Wii Fit, Dance Dance revolution). The class size ranged from 18 to 24. The inclusion criteria were children who: 1) were between 8 and 12 year-olds; 2) had no history of cognitive disabilities in school records; and 3) provided verbal assent and had parental/caregiver consent to participate in the study. Reasons for the inclusion criteria were: 1) children in this age range are able to understand and play exergames; and 2) they were considered to be in an important stage in life where they develop physical activity habits. The study was approved by the University Institutional Review Board and the school district.

Outcome Measures

A standardized questionnaire was used to measure perceived exergaming skills and perceived competence in playing the exergames. Children's perceived exergaming skills variable was assessed by one self-reported question designed specifically for this study. The question asked "How good are you at playing the exergames?" A 5- point Likert scale (1= *not good at all*, 5= *very good*) was used for this measure. To measure situational specific perceived competence, three items from a self-reported questionnaire introduced by Gao, Zhang and Stodden (2013) was adopted. This questionnaire has been demonstrated to be valid and reliable in exergaming

(Gao et al., 2013) and other physical activity settings with this population (Gao, Lee, Kosma, & Solmon, 2010). Specifically, a 5- point Likert scale (1= *strongly disagree*, 5= *strongly agree*) was used to respond to the items with the stem "With regard to the exergaming, I have confidence in…" Sample items were: "my ability to do well in exergaming" and "my ability to learn skills well in exergaming." The mean score of these items was calculated to represent children's perceived competence.

NL-1000 pedometers (New Lifestyles Inc, Lee's Summit, MO) were used to measure children's physical activity level. It has been validated for its accuracy in measuring the level of moderate to vigorous physical activity (Vincent, & Sidman, 2003). Vincent and Sidman's (2003) recommendation was used to validate the pedometers prior to the data collection. Step counts and moderate to vigorous physical activity time were directly retrieved from the outputs, and thus were used as the indicators for children's physical activity in exergaming.

Children's health-related physical fitness was assessed using the 20m Progressive Aerobic Cardiovascular Endurance Run (PACER), curl-ups, and push-ups from the FITNESSGRAM®.[24] FITNESSGRAM tests have demonstrated validity and reliability (Cooper Institute for Aerobic Research, 1999; Morrow, Martin, & Jackson, 2010). Trained research staff completed the testing protocols in a gymnasium or a classroom. The PACER was used to assess cardiovascular fitness and the number of completed laps was recorded and used for data analysis. Muscular strength/endurance was assessed via curl-ups and push-ups. The number of successfully completed repetitions for each test was recorded and used for data analysis.

Procedures

The 50-minute exergaming class was offered to children on a weekly basis at the school throughout 2010-2011. Twelve exergaming stations were set up in a classroom with each station being equipped with various games including, but not limited to, Wii Sports, Wii Fit, and Dance Dance Revolution. No more than two children occupied each game station at a time, and the children rotated to other stations every 15 minutes to experience different kinds of games. Classroom time spent on warm up, cool down, and taking roll limited children's actual exergaming activity time to approximately 35 minutes. A trained physical education teacher was present all the time to oversee the class and help children operate the games. In May 2011, all children responded to a battery of questionnaires measuring their perceived competence and perceived exergaming skills at the end of one exergaming class. Their fitness was then assessed a week later at the gymnasium and their physical activity levels were measured in the following three consecutive weeks (i.e., three exergaming classes). The physical education teacher and the research staff provided instructions and demonstrations for the PACER, push-ups and curl-ups. All children were familiar with all three fitness tests as FITNESSGRAM was the standard fitness testing assessment used by the school district.

Data Analyses

Data were analyzed in three steps. First, Cronbach's alpha coefficients were computed to ensure the internal consistency of the self-report measures. Second, descriptive statistics and Pearson Product Moment Correlations were calculated to describe the sample and evaluate the correlations among the variables. Additionally, structural equation modelling was employed using AMOS 6.0 (Arbuckle, 2003) to test the hypothesized model. Prior to the analysis, the study variables in the model were examined for their normality. Maximum likelihood estimation was used to evaluate the fit of the hypothesized model to the empirical data. Acceptable model fit was assessed using multiple indices. The overall fit of the model to the data was examined via the chi-square divided by degree of freedom. A non-significant chi-square by degree of freedom indicates acceptable model fit (Tabachnick, & Fidell, 2001). Root mean square error of approximation (RMSEA) represents closeness of fit with values approximating 0.06 and zero demonstrating close and exact fit of the model (Hu, & Bentler, 1999). The comparative fit index (CFI), the Tucker-Lewis index (TLI), and the normed fit index (NFI) test the proportionate improvement in fit by comparing the hypothesized model (over identified model) with a just identified model. Acceptable model fit represents CFI, TLI, NFI values higher or equal to 0.95 (Hu, & Bentler, 1999).

RESULTS

Descriptive and Correlation Analyses

The final sample comprised of 236 children (138 boys, 98 girls) due to missing data on one or more outcome variables because of absences on certain data collection days. Cronbach's alpha coefficients for perceived competence were 0.86. The coefficient exceeded the acceptability criterion of 0.70, suggesting that the self-reported perceived competence had acceptable internal consistency. Table 1 shows the means, standard deviations and correlations for all study variables. In general, children scored above the median value on all the self-reported measures since their scores were above the mean of each variable (e.g., 3 for motor skills and perceived competence). Children were physically active in exergaming sessions, with an average of 1058 total steps per session. Children demonstrated large variability on the fitness scores.

Children's perceived exergaming skills, perceived competence, and physical activity levels demonstrated significant, yet low correlations each another (r = 0.17-0.27). Children's physical activity was positively related to PACER (r = 0.15). Additionally, the three components of fitness (PACER, push-up, and curl-up) demonstrated moderate correlations (r = 0.40-0.55).

Table 1. Descriptive Statistics and Correlations among Variables

Variable	Mean	SD	1	2	3	4	5
1. Perceived exergaming skills	4.34	.66	-				
2. Perceived competence	4.00	.75	.24**	-			
3. Physical activity (step)	1058	422	.17**	.27**	-		
4. PACER (lap)	26.02	12.73	-.07	.11	.15**	-	
5. Push-ups (repetition)	11.38	8.21	-.08	.00	.13	.55**	-
6. Curl-ups (repetition)	21.78	14.06	-.09	-.01	.06	.40**	.40**

Notes. SD = Standard Deviation. * $p < .05$; ** $p < .01$.

Mediating Role of Perceived Competence

The hypothesized model demonstrated a good fit to the data, χ^2 (24, N = 244) = 1.218, p = 0.212, CFI = 0.995, TLI = 0.992, NFI = 0.976, RMSEA = 0.025. Figure 1 shows the path diagram and standardized path coefficients of the model. The overall variance (R^2) in perceived competence, physical activity, and fitness explained by the model was 8%, 11% and 3%, respectively. All path coefficients were statistically significant at $p < 0.05$

except for the effect of perceived exergaming skills on physical activity. Perceived exergaming skills had a direct effect on perceived competence (β = 0.29). Perceived competence also had a significant direct effect on physical activity after controlling for the effects of perceived exergaming skills (β = 0.29). However, the direct effect of perceived exergaming skills on physical activity was not significant (β = 0.09). The indirect effect of perceived exergaming skills on physical activity via perceived competence was small, yet significant (β = 0.12). Additionally, physical activity had a direct effect on fitness (β = 0.17). Based on the results, the mediating role of perceived competence on the relations between perceived exergaming skills and physical activity was supported by the hypothesized model.

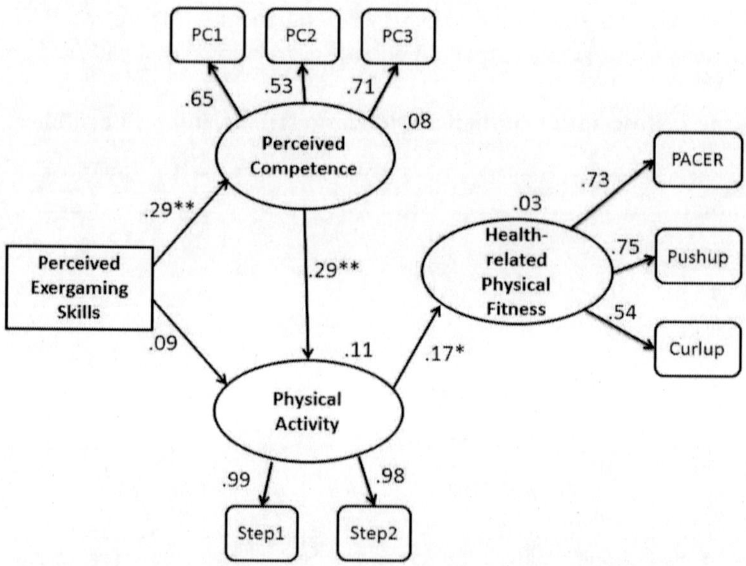

The coefficients on the straight lines are the standardized regression weights; the coefficients above the ovals for PA, perceived competence and fitness are variances explained by the model. **: < .01, * : < .05.

Figure 1. The Mediating Model.

DISCUSSION

This study was the first to examine whether children's perceived competence played a mediating role in the relationships among perceived exergaming skills and physical activity levels in an exergaming setting. Our data suggest that perceived exergaming skills, perceived competence and physical activity were positively related to one another, supporting the first hypothesis. The second hypothesis, postulating that perceived competence, when perceived exergaming skills variable was controlled, had a direct effect on physical activity was supported. This suggests that perceived competence fully mediated the relationship between motor skills and physical activity. The results bolster the Competence Motivation Theory that a child would be more engaged in the behavior if he or she exhibited competence (Harter, 1978). This finding implies that the children who scored higher on perceived competence are more likely to be physically active in exergaming. This is in line with several other studies (Gao, 2008; Skjesol, & Halvari, 2005). For example, Skjesol and Halvari (2005) demonstrated a significant positive correlation between physical activity involvement and perceived sport competence. Gao (2008) also found that situational specific perceived competence explained the variance of physical activity (20.7%) and cardiorespiratory fitness (19.3%) among middle school children. On the other hand, one study reported perceived competence only had a partial mediating effect on relations between motor competence and physical activity (Barnett, Morgan, Van Beurden, Ball, & Lubans, 2011).

In this hypothesized model, the model path between children's perceived exergaming skills did not have a direct effect on physical activity. However, perceived exergaming skills exerted an indirect effect on physical activity via perceived competence, thus supporting its full mediating role. The majority of research findings indicated that there is a positive relation between children's motor skill competence and physical activity (Barnett et al., 2009; Castelli, & Valley, 2007; Fisher et al., 2005; Hume et al., 2008). Only one study suggested that there was no relationship between the two study variables. In particular, in the Kalaja, Jaakkola, Liukkonen, and Watt (2010) study, self-reported physical activity was significantly correlated to perceived competence but not with motor skills (locomotive skills, balance skills and manipulative skill). With the innovative platform of exergaming, children may have been able to enjoy and engage in the various types of exergames, even if they did not possess the skills to perform well. As children were scheduled to rotate stations every 15 minutes, they had the chance to experience various games, which provided them with a higher chance of discovering activities better suited to their preference or proficiency. Thus, exergaming types that offer different skill levels may enable less skillful children to be engaged in the activities. However, this engagement of less skillful children may not always warrant the highest physical activity level, since the beginners' level usually consist of simpler movements. LeGear et al., (2012) found that high perceived competence, in spite of low actual competence, emerges at an early age as young children do not have the cognitive capacity to understand their actual skill. Thus, as participation in many of these games may have been novel for many children, they may not have been able to determine their actual level of skill at a game. And, as winning or losing was not an outcome of these games, children's intrinsic motivation to improve and persist in these types of games may be an important factor as to why perceived competence was associated to perceived exergaming skills and high physical activity participation.

Our data also indicated that physical activity was positively associated with health-related fitness and supports the last hypothesis. The finding is in accordance with previous studies in this line of research (Bürgi et al., 2011; Castelli, & Valley, 2007; Hands, Larkin, Parker, Straker, & Perry, 2009). For instance, Castelli and Valley (2007) found that children's physical activity was significantly related to PACER, curl-ups, push-ups and overall fitness. Hands et al., (2009) also reported that physical activity was positively associated with aerobic fitness. Taken together, the findings imply that the same positive relationships are exhibited in the exergaming setting. That is, actively engaging in exergaming may promote positive changes in health-related physical fitness. The reverse may be true - higher fitness also may allow children to be more physically active for longer periods of time, and hence exploring the mutual effects of physical activity and fitness is warranted in the future.

This study was not without limitations. The first limitation was the use of self-report measure on exergaming skill. While the questionnaire for motor skills is age-appropriate for the children, there is a possibility that children may have overestimated their actual exergaming skill. Second, given the limitation of using pedometers to measure actual physical activity in exergaming, more objective measures of physical activity accelerometers and heart rate monitors would be beneficial.

In addition, it has been evident that boys tend to perform better in the fitness test (Gao, Xiang, Lochbaum, & Guan, 2013). Girls also are likely to play dance games more than boys do in exergaming. Due to the modest sample size, we did not run the model testing for each gender separately in the present study. Further studies may include investigate gender differences of physical activity levels in exergaming play.

CONCLUSION

In summary, these data demonstrated the manner in which children perceived their abilities played a critical role in physical activity engagement in exergaming. Children with a high level of perceived competence are more likely to be physically active than children with low perceived competence. As mentioned previously, it is possible children's judgment about their ability in exergaming is not strongly aligned with their perceived exergaming skill. These results have implications for health educators and practitioners in that positive perception can motivate children to practice for skillfulness and engage in PA. Incorporating fun and enjoyment in programs can be a part of answer. Appropriately designed activities that enhance perceived competence might also promote motivation to learn new skills and keep children engaged.

REFERENCES

Arbuckle, J. L. (2003) *Amos 5.0 Update to the Amos User's Guide*. Chicago, IL: SPSS.

Barnett, L. M., Morgan, P. J., Van Beurden, E., Ball, K., & Lubans, D. R. (2011). A reverse pathway? Actual and perceived skill proficiency and physical activity. *Medicine and Science in Sports and Exercise*, *43*(5), 898–904. doi:10.1249/MSS.0b013e3181fdfadd.

Barnett, L. M., Morgan, P. J., van Beurden, E., & Beard, J. R. (2008). Perceived sports competence mediates the relationship between childhood motor skill proficiency and adolescent physical activity and fitness: A longitudinal assessment. *The International Journal of Behavioral Nutrition and Physical Activity*, *5*, 40. doi:10.1186/1479-5868-5-40.

Barnett, L. M., Van Beurden, E., Morgan, P. J., Brooks, L. O., & Beard, J. R. (2008). Does childhood motor skill proficiency predict adolescent fitness? *Medicine and Science in Sports and Exercise*, *40*(12), 2137–44. doi:10.1249/MSS.0b013e31818160d3.

Barnett, L.M., van Beurden, E., Morgan, P. J., Brooks, L.O., & Beard, J. R. (2009). Childhood motor skill proficiency as a predictor of adolescent physical activity. *Journal of Adolescent Health, 44*(3), 252–259.

Becker, K. (2007). Pedagogy in commercial video games. In D. Gibson, C. Adrich, & M. Prensky, (Eds.), *Games and Simulations in Online*

Learning—Research and development frameworks (pp.21-47). Hershey, PA: Information Science Publishing.

Bürgi, F., Meyer, U., Granacher, U., Schindler, C., Marques-Vidal, P., Kriemler, S., & Puder, J. J. (2011). Relationship of physical activity with motor skills, aerobic fitness and body fat in preschool children: A cross-sectional and longitudinal study (Ballabeina). *International Journal of Obesity (2005), 35*(7), 937–44. doi:10.1038/ijo.2011.54.

Calvert, S. L. (2005). Cognitive effects of video games. In J. Raessens, & F. Goldstein (Eds.), *Handbook of computer game studies* (pp. 125-132). Cambridge, MA: MIT Press.

Castelli, D. M., & Valley, J. A. (2007). Chapter 3 : The Relationship of Physical Fitness and Motor Competence to Physical Activity. *Journal of Teaching in Physical Education*, *26*, 358–374.

Cliff, D. P., Okely, A. D., Smith LM, McKeen, K. (2009). Relationships between fundamental motor skills and objectively measured physical activity in preschool children. *Pediatric Exercise Science, 21*, 436-49.

Cooper Institute for Aerobic Research. (1999). *The FITNESSGRAM Test Administration Manual (2nd ed.)*; Champaign, IL: Human Kinetics.

Fisher, A., Reilly, J.J., Kelly, L. A., Montgomery, C., Williamson, A., Paton, J., & Grant, S. (2005). Fundamental motor skills and habitual physical activity in young children. *Medicine & Science in Sports & Exercise, 37*(4), 684-688.

Gao, Z. (2008). Perceived competence and enjoyment in predicting students' physical activity and cardiorespiratory fitness. *Perceptual and Motor Skills*, *107*, 365-372.

Gao, Z. (2013). The impact of an exergaming intervention on urban school children's physical activity levels and academic outcomes. *Asian Journal of Exercise and Sport Science*, *10*(2), 1–10.

Gao, Z., Hannan, P., Xiang, P., Stodden, D. F., Valdez, V. E. (2013) Video game-based exercise, Latino children's physical health, and academic achievement. *American Journal of Preventive Medicine, 44*(3), S240–246.

Gao, Z., Huang, C., Liu, T., & Xiong, W. (2012). Impact of interactive dance games on urban children's physical activity correlates and behavior. *Journal of Exercise Science & Fitness, 10*(2), 107–112.

Gao, Z., Lee, A. M., Kosma, M., & Solmon, M. (2010). Understanding students' motivation in middle school physical education: examining the mediating role of self-efficacy on physical activity. *International Journal of Sport Psychology*, *41*, 199–215.

Gao, Z., Xiang, P., Lochbaum, M., & Guan, J. (2013). The impact of achievement goals on cardiorespiratory fitness: Does self-Efficacy make a difference? *Research Quarterly for Exercise and Sport*, *84*(3), 313–322. doi:10.1080/02701367.2013.814908.

Gao, Z., Zhang, T., & Stodden, D. (2013). Children's physical activity levels and psychological correlates in interactive dance versus aerobic dance. *Journal of Sport and Health Science*, *2*(3), 146–151. doi:10.1016/j.jshs.2013.01.005

Gunter, B. (2005). Psychological effects of video games. In J. Raessens, & F. Goldstein (Eds.), *Handbook of computer game studies* (pp. 145-160). Cambridge, MA: MIT Press.

Hands, B., Larkin, D., Parker, H., Straker, L., & Perry, M. (2009). The relationship among physical activity, motor competence and health-related fitness in 14-year-old adolescents. *Scandinavian Journal of Medicine & Science in Sports*, *19*(5), 655–63. doi:10.1111/j.1600-0838.2008.00847.x

Harter, S. (1078). Effectance motivation reconsidered: Toward a developmental model. *Human Development, 21*, 34-64.

Hu, L., & Bentler, P. M. (1999). Cutoff criteria for fit indexes in covariance structure analysis: Conventional criteria versus new alternatives. *Structural Equation Modeling*, *6*, 1-55.

Hume, C., Okley, A., Bagley, S., Telford, A., Booth, M., Crawford, D., & Salmon, J. (2008). Does weight status influence associations between children's fundamental movement skills and physical activity? *Research Quarterly for Exercise and Sport*, *79*(2), 158–165.

Kalaja, S., Jaakkola, T., Liukkonen, J., & Watt, A. (2010). Fundamental movement skills and motivational factors influencing engagement in physical activity 1. *Perceptual and Motor Skills*, *111*(1), 115–128. doi:10.2466/06.10.25.PMS.111.4.115-128.

LeGear, M., Greyling, L., Sloan, E., Bell, R. I., Williams, B.-L., Naylor, P.-J., & Temple, V. A. (2012). A window of opportunity? Motor skills and perceptions of competence of children in kindergarten. *The International Journal of Behavioral Nutrition and Physical Activity*, *9*(1), 29. doi:10.1186/1479-5868-9-29.

Lubans, D. R., Morgan, P. J., Cliff, D. P., Barnett, L. M., & Okley, A. (2010). Fundamental movement skills in children and adolescents. *Sports Medicine*, *40*(12), 1019–1035.

Maloney, A. E., Stempel, A., Wood, M. E., Patraitis, C., & Beaudoin, C. (2012). Can dance exergames boost physical activity as a school-based intervention? *Games for Health Journal*, *1*(6), 416–421.

Marshall, J., & Bouffard, M. (1997).The effects of quality daily physical education on movement competency in obese versus non-obese children. *Adaptive Physical Activity Quarterly, 14*, 222-37.

Miller, T., Vaux-Bjerke, A., McDonnell, K., & DiPietro, L. (2013). Can e-gaming be useful for achieving recommended levels of moderate- to vigorous-intensity physical activity in inner-city children? *Games for Health Journal, 2* (2), 96–102.

Morrow, J. R., Martin, S. B., & Jackson, A. W. (2010). Reliability and validity of the FITNESSGRAM: Quality of teacher-collected health-related fitness surveillance data. *Research Quarterly for Exercise & Sport, 81*(3), S24-30.

Okely, A. D., Booth, M. L., & Patterson, J. W. (2001). Relationship of physical activity to fundamental motor skills among adolescents. *Medicine & Science in Sports & Exercise, 33*, 1899-1904.

Peng, W., Crouse, J.C., Lin, J-H. (2013). Using active video games for physical activity promotion: a systematic review of the current state of research. *Health Education & Behavior, 40*(2), 171–192.

Skjesol, K., & Halvari, H. (2005). Motivational climate, achievement goals, perceived sport competence, and involvement in physical activity: Structural and mediator models. *Perceptual and Motor Skills, 100,* 497–523.

Stodden, D. F., Goodway, J. D., Langendorfer, S. J., Roberton, M. A., Rudisill, M. E., Garcia, C., & Garcia, L. E. (2008). A developmental perspective on the role of motor skill competence in physical activity: An emergent relationship. *Quest*, *60*(2), 290–306. doi:10.1080/ 00336297. 2008.10483582

Tabachnick, B. G., & Fidell, L. S. (2001). *Using Multivariate Statistics (4th ed.).* Needham Heights, MA: Allyn & Bacon.

Vedul-Kjelsås, V., Sigmundsson, H., Stensdotter, a-K., & Haga, M. (2012). The relationship between motor competence, physical fitness and self-perception in children. *Child: Care, Health and Development*, *38*(3), 394–402. doi:10.1111/j.1365-2214.2011.01275.x

Vincent, S. D., & Sidman, C. L. (2003). Determining measurement error in digital pedometers. *Measuremen in Physical Education and Exercise Science*, *7*(1), 19–24.

World Health Organization. (2013). *Global strategy on diet, physical activity and health 2013*. Retrieved from http://www.who.int/dietphysicalactivity/ childhood_why/en/index.html

In: Physical Activity Behaviors ...
Editors: Zan Gao and Zachary Pope
ISBN: 978-1-63483-635-7

Chapter 8

ADOLESCENTS' ACCELEROMETER-DETERMINED PHYSICAL ACTIVITY LEVELS IN PHYSICAL EDUCATION: GENDER AND GRADE DIFFERENCES

Zachary Pope and Zan Gao*
University of Minnesota-Twin Cities, Minneapolis, MN, US

ABSTRACT

This study examined whether middle school students' objectively-determined moderate-to-vigorous physical activity in physical education differed by gender and grade in addition to identifying whether students' moderate-to-vigorous physical activity engagement during physical education met the recommended 50% of lesson time. One-hundred forty-seven 6th, 7th, and 8th grade students (75 boys, 72 girls; $Mean_{age}$ = 12.4 years ± 0.99) from a public school in the Southern region of the United States participated in the study. The physical education classes consisted of tag games during the data collection period. Student's percentage of time spent in moderate-to-vigorous physical activity during physical education and average counts per minute in moderate-to-vigorous physical activity were measured by Actical accelerometers. Descriptive analyses were conducted after which a 2 gender x 3 grade multivariate

* Corresponding Author address: 207 Cooke Hall, 1900 University Ave. SE, Minneapolis, MN, 55455, Email: gaoz@umn.edu

analysis of variance was conducted. Descriptive analyses revealed that the participants were physically active. A 2 gender x 3 grade multivariate analysis of variance yielded a significant interaction effect ($p < .01$) and a main effect for grade (p <0 .01). Specifically, our data indicated 6th grade boys spent the highest percentage of physical education time in moderate-to-vigorous physical activity compared to all other grades regardless of gender, whereas 7th grade girls were the least active in comparison to all genders in all other grades. Unexpectedly, 8th grade girls demonstrated a higher percentage of time in moderate-to-vigorous physical activity during physical education than the 6th and 7th grade girls and the 7th and the 8th grade boys. Further research with qualitative methodology (e.g., interviews, focus groups) is warranted to explore this phenomenon.

Keywords: accelerometer, moderate-to-vigorous physical activity, tag games

INTRODUCTION

Low physical activity in youth has contributed to the recent increase in the obesity prevalence and the onset of cardiovascular disease risk factors (Carnethon, Gulati, & Greenland, 2005; Hedley et al., 2004). Obesity is the most significant predictor of hypertension, diabetes, cardiovascular and coronary heart disease, and is associated with abnormal lipid profiles during childhood and adolescence (Dietz, 1998; Styne, 2001). Further, previous studies indicate overweight/obese in youth to be a strong predictor of adult obesity (Must, 1996; Styne, 2001). Regular engagement in moderate-to-vigorous physical activity during physical education class and everyday activities reduces the incidence of overweight, diabetes and other chronic health diseases while also assisting youth in the establishment and maintenance of a healthy lifestyle (Ballard et al., 2005). Despite the aforementioned health benefits, physical activity continues to decline in youth due to the current prevalence of sedentary lifestyles among this population (Sirard, Kubik, Fulkerson, & Arcan, 2008; Strong et al., 2005; Parish & Treasure, 2003). Presently, many children and youth spend large amounts of time playing video games and watching TV. Research has shown that youth spend more than four hours per day watching TV and playing video games with a majority of these youth not meeting physical activity recommendations (Jordan, Hersey, McDivitt, & Heitzler, 2006).

Physical education provides unique opportunities to promote healthful PA behavior changes in school-age youth (National Association for Sports and

Physical Education, 2004; Pate et al., 2006; Sallis & McKenzie, 1991). Intervention studies among school-age youth suggest that the type, duration, frequency, and intensity of physical activity are important and variable determinants of specific health and fitness benefits (Strong et al., 2005). A comprehensive review recommends that all school-age youth engage daily in at least 60 minutes of moderate-to-vigorous physical activity that is enjoyable and developmentally appropriate (Strong et al., 2005).

In addition, students' moderate-to-vigorous physical activity participation in physical education classes is recommended to comprise at least 50% of class time (Pate et al., 2006; U.S. Department of Health and Human Services, 2000). Despite these recommendations, evidence has shown that students in physical education spend a great deal of time being inactive and that current recommendations for moderate-to-vigorous physical activity during physical education are not being met (Fairclough & Stratton, 2005; Grunbaum, Kann, Kinchen, Ross, Hawkins, & Lowry et al., 2004; McKenzie, Marshall, Sallis, & Conway, 2000; Sallis & McKenzie, 1991; Simons-Morton, Taylor, Snider, Huang, & Fulton 1994; U.S. Department of Health and Human Services, 2000).

A study reported that middle school-age youth engaged in moderate-to-vigorous physical activity only 37% of the physical education class duration (Coviello & Dyson, 2005). Another study, using direct observations in secondary physical education classes, showed that students spent 24% of the time participating in moderate-to-vigorous physical activity during physical education (Simon-Morton et al., 1994) which, again, is far below the recommended amounts of moderate-to-vigorous physical activity participation for physical education.

Researchers (e.g., Kulinna et al., 2003; Stratton, 1997; Vincent & Pangrazi, 2002) have also reported grade and age differences in relation to physical activity levels during physical education classes. Inconclusive findings have been reported for students' moderate-to-vigorous physical activity levels as a function of gender. Mckenzie and colleagues (2000) reported that middle school boys were more physically active than girls regardless of activity type as assessed by the System for Observing Fitness Instruction Time. Additionally, some researchers have reported that boys are likely to be more active in physical education than girls (Fairclough & Stratton, 2005; Lemura, Andreacci, Carlonas, Klebez, & Chelland, 2000; Trost, Saunders, & Ward, 2002 b).

By contrast, other researchers (Kulinna, Martin, Lai, Kliber, & Reed, 2003; Laurson, Brown, Cullen, & Dennis, 2008; Sarkin, McKenzi, & Sallis,

1997) have reported no gender differences in physical activity levels as assessed by heart-rate monitors and accelerometers. Finally, a recent study reported no gender or grade influence on physical activity levels in the high school physical education setting; however, physical activity was strongly associated with activity type (Laurson et al., 2008). These inconsistent results may be due, in particular, to the type of instrument used to assess physical activity, activity type, and/or the characteristics of the study population.

Age-related physical activity declines in recommended amounts of moderate-to-vigorous physical activity have been a public concern in youth (Sallis, Prochaska, & Taylor, 2000; Sirard et al., 2008; Strong et al., 2005; Parish & Treasure, 2003). Indeed, recommended amounts of moderate-to-vigorous physical activity markedly decline with increasing grade levels (Aaron, Storti, Robertson, Kriska, & LaPorte, 2002; Grunbaum et al., 2004; Sirard et al., 2008). Generally, moderate-to-vigorous physical activity begins to decline during middle school (Parish & Treasure, 2003).

Stratton (1997) showed students' moderate-to-vigorous physical activity participation increased between nine to 10 years of age, peaked at 11 to 12 years of age, and then decreased in later school years. A similar study reported physical activity participation in secondary school youth during physical education was lower than elementary school youth (Kulinna et al., 2003). Finally, a recent study designed to examine physical activity patterns in female youth found that participation in vigorous physical activity declined significantly between the 8th and 12th grades (Pate, Dowda, O'Neill, & Ward, 2007).

Given the fact that an important health objective of *Healthy People 2010* is to devote at least 50% of physical education class time to moderate-to-vigorous physical activity participation (U.S. Department of Health and Human Services, 2000), physical education programs represent an important avenue to promote school children's moderate-to-vigorous physical activity levels (National Association for Sport and Physical Education, 2004; Pate et al., 2006).

While evidence suggests children differ in their moderate-to-vigorous physical activity engagement during physical education classes across gender and grade (e.g., Kulinna et al., 2003; Vincent & Pangrazi, 2002), few studies have been conducted to determine children's physical activity participation in physical education as measured by accelerometers with an examination of moderate-to-vigorous physical activity by gender and grade levels. Therefore, the purpose of this study was to objectively assess via accelerometry, whether moderate-to-vigorous physical activity engagement time differed by gender and grade and to identify whether 50% of lesson time in middle school physical education was devoted to moderate-to-vigorous physical activity.

METHODS

Participants

The participants were 147 6th, 7th, and 8th grade students (*M* age = 12.4, *SD* = ± 0.99, age range = 10-14 year; 75 boys, 72 girls) enrolled in one public school in the Southern region of the United States. A majority of the participants in this study were from families of middle to high socioeconomic status with the following self-report ethnic breakdown: White American (*n* = 124), African American (*n* = 14), Hispanic American (*n* = 5), Asian American (*n* = 3), and undeclared (*n* = 1). Permission to conduct this study was obtained from the University Institutional Review Board, the school district, the principal and the physical education teachers. Parental consent and child assent to participate in the study was also obtained prior to the start of the study.

The participants had a 90-minute co-educational physical education class taught by three physical education teachers on alternate days. All three teachers had a masters degree in physical education teacher education, had at least 10 years teaching experience, and shared responsibilities for the teaching of the three classes of each grade. The typical class size was 30 to 35 students. Following students' arrival at the gym, the physical education teachers took roll after which the students participated in warm-up activities. After warm-up and during the class lesson, students were organized for the practice of pertinent game skills and provided feedback when necessary. Classes ended with a review of the activity's components. Classes were held indoors and no formal instructions were given.

Instrumentation

A total of 25 accelerometers were used in this study, allowing most of the participants in a class to be monitored simultaneously. Students reported their gender, race, grade, age, height and weight on a demographic information sheet prior to the start of the study.

Physical Activity Levels. Accelerometers have been widely utilized in physical activity research settings as they are simple to use, minimize subject burden, and classify the intensity and duration of physical activity (Puyau, Adolph, Vohra, Zakeri & Butte, 2004; Sirard & Pate, 2001). The sensitivity of accelerometers allow for identification of various intensities of movement (Puyau et al., 2004). In the current study, water resistant Actical accelerometers were utilized (28 x 27 x 10 mm, 17 g with a watch battery, Mini-Mitter Co., Inc., Bend, OR) during regularly scheduled physical education classes in order to assess students' in-class physical activity levels. Actical devices were programmed and downloaded by connecting the monitor to a serial port computer interface using ActiReaders. Once data were downloaded to the corresponding software, data files were exported to Microsoft Excel (Microsoft Corporation, Redmond, WA).

Actical accelerometers have been found to be valid and reliable when used with youth (Puyau et al., 2004; Pfeiffer, McIver, Dowda, Almeida, & Pate, 2006). Pfeiffer and colleagues (2006) provided strong support for the validation for this instrument, showing a high correlation ($r = 0.89$) between VO_2 and activity counts. Given that longer epochs are unable to capture short periods of high activity counts (Nilsson, Ekelund, Yugve, & Sjostrom, 2002), the Actical monitors were set to a 15-second epoch to better capture short bursts of activity typical of school youth (Pfeiffer et al., 2006). Physical activity levels in this study were quantified as average activity counts per minute (average count/min) for activities of moderate to vigorous intensity. Activity cutoff points established by Puyau et al., (2004) were applied to the data: (a) 0-99 counts per minute = sedentary; (b) 100-1499 counts per minute = light; and (c) $\geq$ 1500 counts per minute = moderate-to-vigorous physical activity. In the current study, students' percentage of time engaged in moderate-to-vigorous physical activity was quantified as the time students engaged in moderate-to-vigorous physical activity divided by the duration of the physical education class (60 minutes; Arnett & Lutz, 2003). This outcome variable, percentage of time in moderate-to-vigorous physical activity, was retrieved directly from the Actical outputs.

Procedures

Data collection took place during within three different physical education classes observed for three days each. Throughout the entire data collection period, curricular activities consisted of several types of tag games with handballs, OMNIKIN kin balls, and softballs. Research staff coordinated a schedule with the physical education teachers for the data collection so as to not interrupt their instructional time. In the present study, one accelerometer was locked to the left side of a waistband before the beginning of class and distributed to students as the teachers took roll. Each student was assigned an identification number which corresponded to the number on his or her accelerometer. Given the time allotted for dress change and roll call, approximately 60 minutes was typically devoted to the physical education lesson. The research staff assisted the students in the correct placement of the accelerometers around their waists (i.e., left side) and recorded the class start and end times to ensure identical time frames for subsequent data analysis.

Data Analyses

Descriptive analyses were used to examine the students' percentage of moderate-to-vigorous physical activity time per class, using means and standard deviation. A 2 gender x 3 grade multivariate analysis of variance was performed to examine whether students' percentages of time in moderate-to-vigorous physical activity and average counts in moderate-to-vigorous physical activity differed by gender and grade in middle school physical education. Statistical significance was $\alpha = 0.05$. All statistical analyses were performed using SPSS statistical software, version 15.0 (SPSS Inc., Chicago, IL).

RESULTS

Table 1 shows the percentage of time engaged in moderate-to-vigorous physical activity per class by gender and grade for the whole sample.

Descriptive analyses revealed that participants were sufficiently physically active in their classes (i.e., $Mean_{\%} = 63.22 \pm 13.37$, $Mean_{counts} = 4762.89 \pm 965.92$), as percentages of class time engaged in moderate-to-vigorous physical activity were greater than 50%. A 2 gender x 3 grade multivariate analysis of variance yielded a significant interaction effect (Wilks' Lambda = 0.90, F (4, 280) = 3.80, $p < 0.01$, $\eta^2 = 0.05$) and a main effect by grade (Wilks' Lambda = 0.82, F (4, 280) = 7.49, $p < 0.01$, $\eta^2 = 0.10$). The percentage of moderate-to-vigorous physical activity time were found to be significantly higher than the recommended 50% in the 6th grade boys (75.3%), followed by

Table 1. Percentage of MVPA Time Engagement for Boys (N = 75) and Girls (N = 72)

Boys (N = 75)	Grade	Mean (%)	SD	N	Girls (N = 72)	Grade	Mean (%)	SD	N
Time in Sedentary	6th	6.29	4.56	22		6th	8.45	7.23	27
	7th	11.59	6.18	25		7th	13.47	6.21	24
	8th	5.99	7.42	28		8th	1.14	1.37	21
	Total	7.94	6.72	75		Total	7.99	7.50	72
Time in Light Intensity	6th	18.41	7.47	22		6th	29.62	10.65	27
	7th	30.93	13.27	25		7th	32.08	12.05	24
	8th	30.46	9.99	28		8th	30.12	10.39	21
	Total	27.08	11.87	75		Total	30.59	10.96	72
Time in Moderate-to-Vigorous Intensity	6th	75.29	7.86	22		6th	61.91	12.02	27
	7th	57.46	12.41	25		7th	54.44	12.51	24
	8th	63.54	13.33	28		8th	68.73	10.85	21
	Total	64.96	13.56	75		Total	61.41	13.00	72

Note. SD = Standard Deviation: N = number of the participants: MV = moderate to vigorous.

the 8th grade girls (68.3%) and the 8th grade boys (63.5%). Additionally, we also found students' percentage of class time engaged in moderate-to-vigorous physical activity at different grade levels was affected by gender with the exception being the comparison between 8th grade boys and girls.

Notably, 8th grade girls showed relatively high activity counts and percentage of moderate-to-vigorous physical activity duration per class. By contrast, the 7th grade boys and girls showed the lowest activity counts and percentage of moderate-to-vigorous physical activity per class among all grades and genders.

DISCUSSION

The main purpose of this study was to examine whether middle school students engaged in moderate-to-vigorous physical activity for at least 50% of physical education lesson time as recommended by *Healthy People 2010*. Findings indicate a majority of the students met or exceeded the 50% recommendation when moderate-to-vigorous physical activity and physical activity intensity was assessed via accelerometers. Data revealed that boys were more active than girls (65% vs. 61%, respectively) based on the mean percentage of class time engaged in moderate-to-vigorous physical activity—a finding consistent with many previous studies (Caseprsen et al., 2000; Laurson et al., 2008; Lemura et al., 2000; Mckenzie et al., 2000; Trost, Pate, Sallis, Freedson, Taylor, & Dowd et al., 2002 a). Further, physical activity has consistently demonstrated faster decline among girls compared to boys as boys are more likely to be active and to engage in more moderate-to-vigorous physical activity (Caspersen, Pereria, & Curran, 2000; Centers for Disease Control and Prevention, 2006; Trost et al., 2002 a). Moreover, a recent study reported that only 39.4% and 29.1% of a 50-minute physical education lesson were spent in moderate-to-vigorous physical activity among boys and girls, respectively (Fairclough & Stratton, 2005) based on the recommendation that 50% of lesson time be comprised of moderate-to-vigorous physical activity (U.S. Department of Health and Human Services, 2000; Pate et al., 2006). However, the results of the current study indicated that playing tag games facilitated the recommended percentage of moderate-to-vigorous physical activity time during physical education classes. Therefore, the findings of this study substantiate the recommendations that 50% of the physical education time should involve moderate-to-vigorous physical activity.

With respect to the grade effect, younger boys spent the highest percentage of time in moderate-to-vigorous physical activity compared to all other grades regardless of gender, whereas the 7th grade girls were the least active in comparison to all genders and grades. Unexpectedly, 8th grade girls demonstrated a higher percentage of time in moderate-to-vigorous physical activity than the 6th and 7th grade girls and the 7th and the 8th grade boys. The reason for the differences found in our study is not well understood and deserves further investigation.

Additionally, many factors are related to students' active participation in moderate-to-vigorous physical activity during physical education. A recent study reported that gender and grade were not associated with physical activity levels in the high school physical education setting (Laurson et al., 2008). However, Laurson and colleagues (2008) found a significant relationship between physical activity level and type of activity, indicating that girls spent more time in individual activities than boys while boys engaged more in team sports than girls. In addition, another study reported that elementary school youth showed the highest physical activity levels, followed by high school and middle school youth (Kulinna et al., 2003). Further, a recent study designed to examine physical activity patterns in female youth found that participation in vigorous physical activity declined significantly between 8th and 12th grades. Yet, researchers found that the probability of participation in vigorous forms of PA in the 12th grade was strongly associated with participation in vigorous forms of physical activity in the 8th grade (Pate et al., 2007). A similar study reported that cardiorespiratory fitness in female students changed from middle to high school, declining from 9th to 12th grades (Pfeiffer, Dowda, Dishman, Sirard, & Pate, 2007). This study suggested that active sport participation and physical activity in female students should be encouraged to maintain cardiorespiratory fitness level in high school (Pfeiffer et al., 2007).

Several studies have also reported a relationship between moderate-to-vigorous physical activity and body fatness (Butte, Puyau, Adolph, Vohra, & Zakeri, 2007; Patrick et al., 2004) wherein increasing body fatness is strongly associated with declining physical activity. Specifically, the aforementioned study indicate that increasing body fatness is strongly associated with declining physical education experience and other pertinent characteristics of the study population (e.g., overweight status, previous sport participation, level of students' physical fitness, student motivation, & teacher impact). Lastly, students' enjoyment of physical education (Sallis, Prochaska, Taylor, Hill, & Geraci, 1999), student motivation, and poor teaching skills and practices are strongly associated with level of physical activity (Simons-Morton et al.,

1994). To build upon the findings of the current study and the knowledge gaps among the literature, future research might use surveys measuring students' attitudes and motivation coupled with in-depth interview or focus groups. This may help explain the mixed findings among physical activity levels, gender and grade. In addition, it was beyond the scope of this current study to determine the predictors of low moderate-to-vigorous physical activity. Future study is needed to determine the cause of low moderate-to-vigorous physical activity time engagement in physical education. For instance, students' body fatness, which can affect percentage of moderate-to-vigorous physical activity engagement time in physical education, could be assessed using a simple field measure (e.g., body mass index and/or waist circumference).

In conclusion, our data suggested that younger boys spent the highest percentage of physical education time in moderate-to-vigorous physical activity whereas 7th grade students, especially girls, were not as active as other grades. Nonetheless, the findings also suggest the physical education classes in this study met the currently recommended moderate-to-vigorous physical activity amounts and provide interesting empirical evidence for middle school students' moderate-to-vigorous physical activity in physical education of which contrasts with many previously literature. Physical education must be a part of school curriculum for all students, because physical education provides students with moderate-to-vigorous physical activity engagement while also teaching them to make informed decisions on how to achieve and maintain a physically active lifestyle now and throughout their life. However, physical activity participation in secondary school physical education has been declining with respect to physical education enrollment and the number of physical education classes each week (Lowry & Wechsler, Kann, & Collins, 2001). Reduced physical education class time limits the impact schools have on youth to become a physically educated person (National Association for Sport and Physical Education, 2004). In a recent cross-sectional study including 878 youth aged 11-15 years, it was reported that 55% of youth failed to meet physical activity guidelines (Sanchez, Norman, Sallis, Calfas, Cella, & Patrick, 2007). Therefore, it is important that schools provide an adequate amount of physical education time and quality physical education programs for all genders and ages—especially when one considers that for youth of lower socioeconomic status physical education may be the only time of the day that they get to participate in organized and supervised physical activity. For instance, providing students with opportunities to learn how to implement some simple physical activity tools (e.g., 3 Day Physical Activity log & pedometer activity) and to teach them how to monitor moderate-to-vigorous physical activity in physical education can motivate students to be more active as they assume responsibility for their own activity choices in and outside of physical education class (Oh & Hovatter, 2010).

More studies are needed to identify and develop practical strategies to increase physical activity through school physical education with the current study suggesting a particular emphasis on 7th grade girls. In addition, the current study included only one school. Therefore, future studies need to recruit a large number of diverse students from multiple school sites to increase the generalizability of the findings. Finally, future studies need to include various activity units to examine students' moderate-to-vigorous physical activity engagement time in physical education in order to confirm the findings from the present investigation.

REFERENCES

Aaron, D.J., Storti, K.L., Robertson, R.J., Kriska, A.M., & LaPorte, R.E. (2002). Longitudinal study of the number and choice of leisure time physical activities from mid to late adolescence. *Archives of Pediatric & Adolescent Medicine, 156,* 1075-1080.

Arnett, M.C., & Lutz, R.B. (2003). Measurement of moderate to vigorous physical activity of middle school girls, using Tritrac activity monitors during small-sided, game-based lessons. *Measurement in Physical Education & Exercise Science, 7,* 149-159.

Ballard, K., Caldwell, D., Dunn, C., Hardison, A., Newkirk, J., Sanderson, M., Thaxton, V.S., & Thomas, C. (2005). *Move more, NC's Recommended Standards for Physical Activity in School.* North Carolina Department of Health and Human Services, NC Division of Public Health, Raleigh, NC.

Butte, N.F., Cai, G., Cole, S.A., & Comuzzie, A.G. (2006). Viva la Familia Study: Genetic and environmental contributions to childhood obesity and its comorbidities in the Hispanic population. *American Journal of Clinical Nutrition, 84,* 646-654.

Carnethon, M.R., Gulati, M., & Greenland, P. (2005). Prevalence and cardiovascular disease correlates of low cardiorespiratory fitness in adolescents and adults. *Journal of the American Medical Association, 294*, 2981-2988.

Caspersen, C.J., Pereria, M.A., & Curran, K.M. (2000). Changes in physical activity patterns in the United States, by gender and cross-sectional age. *Medicine & Science in Sports & Exercise*, *32*, 1601-1609.

Coviello, N., & Dyson, B. (2005). Middle school students' physical activity levels and students' perspectives in the gymnasium. *Research Quarterly for Exercise and Sport*, 76, A-68.

Dietz, W.H. (1998). Health consequences of obesity in youth: Childhood predictors of adult disease. *Pediatrics, 101*, 518-525.

Fairclough, S. J., & Stratton, G. (2005). Physical education makes you fit and healthy: Physical education's contribution to young people's physical activity levels. *Health Education Research, 20*, 14-23.

Grunbaum, J.A., Kann, L., Kinchen., S., Ross, J., Hawkins, J., & Lowry, R. (2004). Youth Risk Behaviors Surveilance-United States, 2003, *Morbility and Mortality Weekly Report, 53,* 1-29.

Hedley, A.A., Ogden, C.L., Johnson, C.L., Carroll, M.D., Curtin, L.R., & Flegal, K.M. (2004). Prevalence of overweight and obesity among US children, adolescents, and adults, 1999-2002. *Journal of the American Medical Association, 291*, 2847- 2850.

Jordan, A.B., Hersey, J.C., McDivitt, J.A., & Heitzler, C.D. (2006). Reducing children's television-viewing time: A qualitative study of parents and their children. *Pediatrics, 118,* 1303-1310.

Kulinna, P.H., Martin, J., Lai, Q., Kliber, A., & Reed, B. (2003). Student physical activity patterns: Grade, gender and activity influences. *Journal of Teaching in Physical Education, 22*, 298-310.

Laurson, K.R., Brown, D.D., Cullen, R.W., & Dennis, K.K. (2008). Heart rates of high school physical education students during team sports, individual sports, and fitness activities. *Research Quarterly for Exercise and Sport, 79,* 85-91.

Lemura, L., Andreacci, J., Carlonas, R., Klebez, J., & Chelland, S. (2000). Evaluation of physical activity measured via accelerometry in rural fourth-grade children. *Perceptual and Motor Skills, 90*, 329-337.

Lowry, R., Wechsler, H., Kann, L., & Collins, J.L. (2001). Recent trends in participation in physical education among U.S. high school students. *Journal of School Health, 71,* 145-152.

McKenzie, T.L., Marshall, S.J., Sallis, J.F., & Conway, T.L. (2000). Student activity levels, lesson context, and teacher behavior during middle school physical education. *Research Quarterly for Exercise and Sport, 71,* 249-259.

Must, A. (1996). Morbidity and mortality associated with elevated body weight in children and adolescents. *American Journal of Clinical Nutrition, 63*, 445-447.

National Association for Sport and Physical Education. (2004). *Moving into future: National standards for physical education*. Reston, VA: National Association for Sport and Physical Education.

Nilsson, A., Ekelund, U., Yngve, A., & Sjöstrom, M. (2002). Assessing physical activity among children with accelerometers during different time sampling intervals and placements. *Pediatric Exercise Science, 14,* 87-96.

Oh, H., & Hovatter, R. (2010). Monitoring moderate to vigorous physical activity in high school physical education. *Future Focus, 31*(1), 18-25.

Parish, L.E., & Treasure, D.C. (2003). Physical activity and situational motivation in physical education: Influence of the motivational climate and perceived ability. *Research Quarterly for Exercise and Sport, 74*, 173-182.

Pate, R.R., Ward, D.S., O'Neill, J.R., & Dowda, M. (2007). Enrollment in physical education is associated with overall physical activity in adolescent girls. *Research Quarterly for Exercise and Sport*, *78*, 265-270.

Pate, R.R., Davis, M.G., Robinson, T.N., Stone, E.J., McKenzie, T.L., & Young, J.C. (2006). Promoting physical activity in children and youth a leadership for schools: A scientific Statement from the American Heart Association Council on nutrition, physical activity, and metabolism (physical activity committee) in collaboration with the councils on cardiovascular disease in the young cardiovascular nursing. *Circulation, 114*, 1214-1224.

Patrick, K., Norman, G.J., Calfas, K.J., Sallis, J.F., Zabinski, M.F., Rupp, J., et al., (2004). Diet, physical activity, and sedentary behaviors as risk factors for overweight in adolescence. *Archives of Pediatrics & Adolescent Medicine, 158,* 385-390.

Pfeiffer, K., McIver, K., Dowda, M., Almeida, J., & Pate, R. (2006). Validity and calibration of the Actical accelerometer in preschool children. *Medicine & Science in Sports & Exercise, 38*(1), 152-157.

Pfeiffer, K., Dowda, M., Dishman, R.K., Sirard, J.R., & Pate, R. (2006). Cardiorespiratory fitness in girls.-change from middle to high school *Medicine & Science in Sports & Exercise, 39*(12), 2234-2241.

Puyau, M.R., Adolph, A.L., Vohra, F.A., Zakeri, I., & Butte, N.F. (2004). Prediction of activity energy expenditure using accelerometers in children. *Medicine Science in Sport & Exercise*, *36*, 1625-1631.

Sallis, J.F., & McKenzie,T.L. (1991). Physical education's role in public health. *Research Quarterly for Exercise and Sport, 64,* 25-31.

Sallis, J.F., Prochaska, J.J., Taylor, W.C., Hill, J.O., & Geraci, J.C. (1999). Correlates of physical activity in a national sample of girls and boys in grades four through twelve. *Health Psychology, 18,* 410-415.

Sallis, J.F., Prochaska, J.J., & Taylor, W.C. (2000). A review of correlates of physical activity of children and adolescents. *Medicine & Science in Sports & Exercise, 32*, 963-975.

Sanchez, A., Norman, G.J., Sallis, J.F., Calfas, K.J., Cella, J., & Patrick, K. (2007). Patterns and correlates of physical activity and nutrition behaviors in adolescents. *American Journal of Preventive Medicine, 32*, 124-130.

Sarkin, J.A., McKenzie, T.L., & Sallis, J.F. (1997). Gender differences in physical activity during fifth-grade physical education and recess periods. *Journal of Teaching in Physical Education, 17,* 99-106.

Simons-Morton, B.G., Taylor, W.C., Snider, S.A., Huang, I.W., & Fulton, J.E. (1994). Observed levels of elementary and middle school children's physical activity during physical education classes. *Preventive medicine, 23*, 437-441.

Sirard, J.R., Kubik, M.Y., Fulkerson, J.A., & Arcan, C. (2008). Objectively measured physical activity in urban alternative high school students. *Medicine in Science & Sports & Exercise, 40,* 2088-2095.

Sirard, J.R., & Pate, R.R. (2001). Physical activity assessment in children and adolescents. *Sports Medicine, 31,* 439-454.

Stratton, G. (1997). Children's heart rates during British physical education lessons. *Journal of Teaching in Physical Education, 16*, 357-367.

Strong, W.B., Malina, R.M., Blimkie, C.J., Daniels, S.R., Dishman, R.K., Gutin, B,...Trudeau, F. (2005). Evidence based physical activity for school-age youth. *Journal of Pediatrics, 146*, 732-737.

Styne, D. M. (2001). Childhood and adolescent obesity: Prevalence and significance. *Pediatric Clinics of North American, 48*(4), 823-854.

Trost, S.G., Pate, R.R., Sallis, J.F., Freedson, P.S., Taylor, W.C., Dowda, M., & Sirard, J. (2002a). Age and gender differences in objectively measures physical activity in youth. *Medicine & Science in Sports & Exercise, 34*, 350–355.

Trost, S.G., Saunders, R., & Ward, D.S. (2002 b). Determinants of physical activity in middle school children. *American Journal of Health Behavior, 26,* 95-102.

U.S. Department of Health and Human Services. (2000). *Healthy people 2010:Understanding and improving health.* Washington, DC: U.S. Government Printing Office.

Vincent, S.D., & Pangrazi, R.P. (2002). An examination of the activity patterns of elementary school children. *Pediatric Exercise Science, 14,* 432-441.

In: Physical Activity Behaviors …
Editors: Zan Gao and Zachary Pope
ISBN: 978-1-63483-635-7

Chapter 9

PHYSICAL ACTIVITY AND CARDIOVASCULAR FITNESS IN PHYSICAL EDUCATION: THEORETICAL CORRELATES AND MODERATORS

***You Fu*[1], *Zan Gao*[2], *Ryan D. Burns*[3] *and James C. Hannon*[4]**

[1]University of Nebraska Kearney, Kearney, NE, US
[2]University of Minnesota-Twin Cities, Minneapolis, MN, US
[3]University of Utah, Salt Lake City, UT, US
[4]West Virginia University, Morgantown, WV, US

ABSTRACT

Previous studies that aimed to explore children and adolescents' psychomotor and socio-motivational variables in school physical education settings have indicated that middle and high school students do not achieve sufficient levels of moderate-to-vigorous physical activity. It has also been documented that the pediatric population often lacks motivation to participate in active play on a regular basis. This review examined published studies that explored the factors correlated with adolescents' physical activity and health-related fitness levels. The review revealed that students' physical activity participation and cardiovascular fitness levels are influenced by motivational beliefs (enjoyment and perceived competence), significant others, gender, and age. The findings suggest that a better understanding of the relationships and interactive associations of those influential factors in physical education is needed in order to increase children and adolescents' moderate-to-vigorous physical activity and cardiovascular fitness levels.

Keywords: enjoyment, health-related fitness, motivation, perceived competence

INTRODUCTION

The health of American children is a major public concern with obesity rates steadily increasing in prevalence (Robinson, Yardy, & Carter, 2012; Welk & Blair, 2000). This is due, in part, to low levels of physical activity and an increase in sedentary behaviors such as TV watching and video games (U.S. Department of Health & Human Services [USDHHS], 2008; 2001). Sedentary habits and low physical fitness levels in adolescents can track into adulthood, which has potentially significant consequences for both individuals and society (Malina, 2007). As a consequence, there has been an increased recognition of the importance of optimal levels of physical activity and fitness among children and adolescents. Indeed, numerous research studies have been conducted on the pediatric population to examine effective strategies to increase healthy behaviors in school settings (McKenzie, 2003; Sallis et al., 1997).

It has been reported that regular physical activity participation has a positive influence on individuals' health and well-being (Roberts & Barnard, 2005). Children and adolescents who participate in optimal levels of physical activity on a daily basis are at a decreased risk of developing early onset chronic diseases such as type II diabetes and cardiovascular disease (Strong et al., 2005). Promoting physical activity and cardiovascular fitness is one of the primary goals of school physical education programs. In response to the link between physical activity and health, it has been recommended by various health agencies that children and adolescents should participate in moderate to vigorous physical activity for at least 60 minutes per day (Biddle, Gorely, & Stensel, 2004; National Association for Sport and Physical Education [NASPE], 2004; Strong et al., 2005).

Despite these recommendations, research indicates 90% of the school children and adolescents do not meet the recommended levels, which may contribute to the increased prevalence in overweight and obesity in this population (Troiano et al., 2008; USDHHS, 2008).

OVERVIEW OF COMPETENCE MOTIVATION THEORY

Researchers have concluded that theory-based interventions are more effective in increasing health-related behaviors compared to non-theoretical interventions (Michie & Abraham, 2004). This is because theories provide a framework to describe the development of interventions as well as offer the resources necessary to evaluate these interventions (The Improved Clinical Effectiveness through Behavioral Research Group, 2006). Motivational beliefs that support optimal levels of physical activity are important for assuring positive health and developmental outcomes. Recently, it has also been reported that there is a positive correlation between motivation and individuals' self-reported physical activity and cardiovascular fitness levels (Gao, Lodewyk, & Zhang, 2009; Martin et al., 2005; Shen, McCaughtry, & Martin, 2007). However, previous research has reported that school children's motivation for physical activity declines as they age into adolescence and early adulthood (Fredricks & Eccles, 2002; Gao, 2009; Jacobs et al., 2002). For example, one longitudinal study aimed to examine the gender and domain differences in perceived competence in 761 children across grades 1 through 12 found a significant decline in children's self-reported perceived sport competence and an accelerated decline across the high school years (Jacobs, Lanza, Osgood, Eccles, & Wigfield, 2002).

Harter (1978) reported several major reasons why youth are motivated to engage in physical activity within the competence motivation theory, which is a helpful resource for determining and predicting what factors inspire individuals to engage in particular activities. Over the past several decades, competence motivation theory has been widely used to investigate students' motivation in sport and physical education settings. The theory proposes that individuals' achievement behaviors can be explained by perceived competence and enjoyment and that individuals tend to be motivated to achieve competence in several achievement fields such as athletics, academics, and peer interactions (Klint & Weiss, 1987). Successfully mastering tasks boosts perceived competence and enjoyment, which, in turn, increases motivated behaviors and performance (Harter, 1981).

According to Harter (1978), there are several major reasons why children are motivated to engage in physical activity. Perceived competence and enjoyment have been identified as significant contributors to physical activity participation and continuous engagement in sport activities (Carroll & Loumidis, 2001; Gao, 2008; Reeve & Weiss, 2006; Weiss & Williams, 2004). As a major construct of motivation, perceived competence is the perception a person has of his or her ability to accomplish certain tasks resulting from cumulative interactions with the environment (Harter, 1985). Perceived competence represents the key idea that most individuals will choose to do a task or continue to engage in a task when they expect to be successful. In particular, children who have higher levels of perceived competence want to develop and demonstrate physical abilities, such as athletic skills and physical fitness.

Researchers have long stated that perceived competence is directly related to physical activity participation motivation (e.g., Chambers, 1991). Several studies have reported a significant positive correlation between students' perceived competence and physical activity levels (Bagoien & Halvari, 2005; Carroll & Loumidis, 2001; Gao, 2008; Kalaja et al., 2010; Stein et al., 2007; Telama, 1998; Williams & Gill, 1995). In a study by Carroll and Loumidis (2001), a sample of 922 British middle school students responded to questionnaires assessing perceived competence regarding their physical education programs. The results suggested that children with higher levels of perceived competence participated in significantly more physical activity (quantity and intensity) outside school compared to those with lower perceived competence. Other studies have also reported a positive correlation between perceived competence and students' health-related physical fitness (Gao, 2008; Gao, Lee, Solmon, & Zhang, 2009). For example, in a study using a sample of 300 middle school students, it was reported that perceived competence was a significant predictor of physical activity and cardiovascular fitness levels (Gao, 2008). Another study also reported that middle school students had higher cardiovascular fitness levels when they believed that they would do well in fitness and physical education (Gao et al., 2009).

In addition to perceived competence, enjoyment is also a dimensional construct of motivation (Wankel, 1997). The concept of enjoyment has been defined as a multidimensional model consisting of factors associated with excitement, affect, competence, attitude, and cognition (Crocker, Bouffard, & Gessaroli, 1995; Wankel, 1997). According to Scanlan and Simons (1992), enjoyment is an important influential factor predicting physical activity participation. Enjoyment derived from physical activity participation maximizes positive and minimizes negative experiences related to the behavior. Therefore, children are more inclined to participate in physical activity if they find it to be enjoyable, and the odds of continued participation will be increased as a result (Kremer, Trew, & Ogle, 1997). Researchers have also suggested that not only is an individual's experience of enjoyment positively associated with physical activity participation (Borra, Schwartz, Spain, & Natchipolsky, 1995), enjoyment is a significant determinant of their participation (Kremer et al., 1997; Wankel, 1993). It has been reported that physical activities providing fun for children are more attractive than boring activities (Craig, Goldberg, & Dietz, 1996; DiLorenzo, Stucky-Ropp, VanderWal, & Gotham, 1998; Sallis & Owen, 1999) with longitudinal studies suggested there was a positive relationship between enjoyment and physical activity during childhood (Shephard & Trudeau, 2000).

To promote positive physical education experiences, the Centers for Disease Control and Prevention (CDC) started recommending that physical education curricula should emphasize student's enjoyment (CDC, 1997). Kalaja et al., (2010) stated that providing enjoyable experiences is a potential strategy for increasing physical activity levels in middle school students and that perceived competence was a significant predictor of physical activity engagement during this process. Wallhead and Buckworth (2004) found that enjoyment in school physical education was related to the motivational factors associated with the adoption of a physically active lifestyle outside school hours. Additionally, enjoyment has been linked with physical activity engagement in school physical education settings (Gao, 2008; Hashim, Grove, & Whipp, 2008; Yli-Piipari, Watt, Jaakkola, Liukkonen, & Nurmi, 2009).

Despite these positive correlations with moderate-to-vigorous physical activity behaviors, enjoyment tends to decline as children age. In a longitudinal study, Prochaska et al., (2003) found a consistent decrease in physical education enjoyment among 4th to 6th grade school children. Similar results were found in another study with Australian 8th grade to 10th grade students during an intervention period of 5 weeks. For grade 8 students, enjoyment levels declined from 82% to 71%, and for grade 10 students enjoyment levels fell from 70% to 62% (Booth et al., 1997). Another study observed Greek students in grades 5, 7, and 10 (Digelidis & Papaioannou, 1999), and confirmed that physical education enjoyment levels were negatively related with the grade level.

Indeed, motivational components of perceived competence and enjoyment have been recognized as the most significant contributors to physical activity participation and continuous engagement in sport activities (Reeve & Weiss, 2006; Weiss & Williams, 2004). It has also been reported that children with higher levels of perceived competence and enjoyment participated in significantly higher physical activity levels (Bell, 1997; Carroll, & Loumidis, 2001; Jacobs et al., 2002; Reeve & Weiss, 2006; Weiss & Williams, 2004). Therefore, researchers must consider both perceived competence and enjoyment when investigating how children's motivation relates to optimal physical activity behaviors and cardiovascular fitness.

MODERATING EFFECTS OF GENDER AND AGE ON PHYSICAL ACTIVITY AND FITNESS

Gender and age are the most powerful determinants in influencing physical activity and fitness levels. In fact, gender and age differences have been frequently reported when studying physical activity and fitness patterns in children and adolescents. The majority of research has suggested boys were more active than girls and that boys had higher self-reported and observed physical activity and physical fitness levels between the ages of 9-13 years (Bois, Sarrazin, Brustad, Trouilloud, & Cury, 2005; Gao, Hannon, Newton, & Huang, 2011; Hobin, Leatherdale, Manske, Dubin, Elliott, & Veugelers, 2012; Hovell, Sallis, Kolody, & Mckenzie, 1999; Kalaja et al., 2010; Kamtsios, 2010; Trost et al., 2002). Additionally, findings from a youth review study suggested a steeper decline in physical activity and physical fitness among girls compared to boys (Sallis, 1993).

In terms of the gender differences seen with regard to motivational beliefs, several studies reported that boys perceived higher levels of perceived competence than girls (Gao et al., 2009; Jacobs et al., 2002), and also tended to have higher enjoyment levels during physical activity than girls (Bois et al., 2005; Gao, Zhang, & Podlog, 2013; Kalaja et al., 2010; Kamtsios, 2010). The aforementioned results are logical given the fact research findings have consistently shown that boys are more likely to demonstrate higher levels of physical activity, cardiovascular fitness, and motivational beliefs in physical education classes.

Unlike age-related changes in academic domains, researchers have documented inconsistent findings for age differences in physical activity levels, physical fitness, and motivational beliefs in physical education settings. The majority of research has reported that children's physical activity and physical fitness levels decline across school years in physical education (Parish & Treasure, 2003; Sallis, 1993, 2000; Trost et al., 2002), whereas some studies have found opposing results. For example, in a 9-year longitudinal study, Telama and his colleagues (Telama & Yang, 2000) indicated that school children's self-reported intensity of physical activity increases with age, especially among boys. Nevertheless, few research studies have been conducted to examine the gender and grade difference in school children's physical fitness levels among various physical education instructional models. This lack of congruence calls for more research.

Moderating Effects of Curricula on Adolescents' Physical Activity and Fitness Levels

Research evidence has shown that various physical education instructional models have different effects on children's physical activity behaviors, cardiovascular fitness, and motivational beliefs (Gao, Zhang, & Podlog, 2013; Spittle & Byrne, 2009; Wallhead & Ntoumanis, 2004). Adolescents' physical activity levels and motivational beliefs have been found to vary in different curricular activities (Fairclough & Stratton, 2006; Gao et al., 2011). Generally, students demonstrate higher physical activity levels during team games, particularly invasion games (e.g., flag football, basketball, and soccer) than health-related fitness activities. MacFarlane and Kwong (2003) found that students demonstrated higher heart rates during ball games and free play than athletics and gymnastics, and direct observation of students' activities further supported that result. However, another study, by Simons-Morton, Taylor, Snider, and Huang (1993) observed that students achieved the most moderate and vigorous intensity of physical activity during walking/jogging, football, and dodge ball, whereas students had the least physical activity intensity during rope climbing and tag games. Another study used accelerometers to evaluate the effects of curricula activity on students' physical activity levels, and reported that students spent a significantly higher percentage of time in moderate-to-vigorous intensity physical activity in fitness and football classes than they did in Dance Dance Revolution classes (Gao et al., 2011).

It has been documented that students' motivation could also be affected by curricular activity (Lee, 1997). For example, perceived competence and enjoyment of the activities emerge as important indicators of students' positive motivation (Gao, 2008; Harter, 1978). However, the potential effect of curricular activities on motivation has been neglected because most motivation-based empirical research concentrated on individuals' psychological temperaments rather than on learner-content reciprocities (Gao et al., 2011). Therefore, examining the relationship between physical education curricular activity and students' motivation toward physical education is imperative.

SPARK was initially designed as a research-based elementary physical education program but now includes preschool, middle school, and high school physical education as well. Considering the prevalence of childhood obesity due, in part, to the poor physical activity participation, the SPARK programs were designed with the objective to increase low levels of children's physical activity and improve cardiovascular fitness (Sallis et al., 1997). It has been reported that present day physical education programs focus more on school children's sport capabilities and that interventions with the aim of promoting children's health-related outcomes need to be designed to promote long-term physical activity participation (Sallis & McKenzie, 1991). Given the aforementioned research, SPARK was developed as a comprehensive school-based physical education program concerned not only with increasing physical activity, but also with promoting the generalization of physical activity and fitness beyond school environments (McKenzie, Sallis, & Rosengard, 2009).

SPARK was developed by the National Heart, Lung, and Blood Institute of the National Institutes of Health and San Diego State University and is a health-oriented physical education program that teaches health activities and behavioral skills to school children (McKenzie, Sallis, & Rosengard, 2009). SPARK curriculum is a comprehensive program designed to promote school students' health-related physical fitness components and promotes students' enjoyment and engagement in physical activity outside of physical education. The curriculum was also designed to promote a moderate to vigorous intensity level of physical activity, health-related fitness, and movement skills. The curriculum package includes yearly plans divided into several instructional units based on various sport activities, each typically 3 to 4 weeks in length. The selection of activities in the SPARK program and the methods employed are designed to promote maximum student participation during class time. The program precludes inactive sports and drills, elimination games, and activities that require specialized and expensive equipment (e.g., swimming class) or demand an inordinate amount of time to set up (Silverman & Ennis, 2003).

A standard lesson of SPARK curriculum includes two parts: activities that focus on health-related physical fitness and those that focus on motor/sport skills. The activities which focus largely on health-related physical fitness are implemented within instructional units which include aerobic dance, aerobic games, and jump rope activities. The intensity, duration, and complexity of these health-related physical fitness activities varies according to different environments but are most focused on developing cardiovascular endurance which, in turn, promotes greater muscular strength and more favorable body composition. Additionally, SPARK has 12 other units concentrating on developing motor skills and age-based skills applied in sport activities such as basketball, soccer, and volleyball. Modifications are also applied to make low-activity games (e.g., softball, kickball) more active. In addition to the physical education curriculum, the SPARK package includes "Lifelong Wellness," which is a self-management program. It aims to help children and adolescents adopt healthy behaviors and skills, and maintain regular physical activity. Finally, practices of self-monitoring, goal setting, self-reinforcement, self-instruction, scheduling, and decision making/problem solving are also included in this instructional package.

A number of publications have demonstrated the positive outcomes of SPARK on school students' in-class physical activity levels, cardiovascular fitness levels, and psychological variables (Fu et al., 2013; Marshall, Biddle, Sallis, McKenzie, & Conway, 2002; McKenzie et al., 2004; McKenzie et al., 2009; Prosper, Moczulski, Quershi, Weiss, & Bryars, 2009; Sallis et al., 2002). Prosper and his colleagues (2009) investigated the effect of SPARK on childhood overweight and obesity and its impact on lifestyle behaviors that promote lifelong fitness and healthy eating habits among 1469 students enrolled in 51 K-12 schools. The study found that body mass index significantly improved among overweight and obese students after the intervention was implemented for 1 school year. Significant improvements were also observed on students' self-esteem scores and indicators for lifestyle behaviors. The study demonstrated that SPARK could help improve the health of low-income families' youth whose neighborhoods are unsafe and often lack exercise facilities. The study further concluded that SPARK provided a safe, accessible, no cost, and effective method in the fight against childhood overweight and obesity.

Other health-oriented school physical education programs have been reported among the literature indicating improvements in children's moderate to vigorous physical activity levels compared to traditional physical education class (McKenzie et al., 1997; McKenzie et al., 2004; Sallis et al., 1997; Sallis et al., 2002). In a study examining the "Go for Health" program, it was found that students in the intervention group displayed significantly higher physical activity levels over 2 years compared to students in the control group (Simons-Morton, Parcel, & O'Hara, 1988). In another experimental study, students in a health-oriented physical education program accumulated higher levels of moderate to vigorous physical activity compared to students in the control group (McKenzie, Sallis, Faucette, Roby, & Kolody, 1993).

LIMITATIONS OF CURRENT LITERATURE

As a result of reviewing previous studies, several common limitations in the research of physical activity and fitness in physical education settings emerged. First, measurement issues still exist in collecting physical activity data in physical education settings. Most of the research used pedometers or systematic observational tools to assess students' physical activity levels with only a small percentage of studies using more valid instruments such as accelerometers. Second, limited research focused on daily physical education curricula as most schools have physical education class only once a week. Therefore, it is difficult to generalize findings regarding the correlates of moderate to vigorous physical activity and health-related fitness levels to daily physical education curricula. Third, most reviewed studies collected data on homogeneous samples of children and adolescents; samples with ethnic diversity should be included in the future studies. Fourth, most of the reviewed studies did not include a long-term follow up to interventions; therefore the sustainability of popular programs to increase moderate to vigorous physical activity and health-related fitness in school settings is questionable. Finally, studies controlling for teachers' years of teaching experience, sex, and educational backgrounds are limited but need to be conducted as these factors may have a significant influence on students' moderate to vigorous physical activity and fitness levels.

IMPLICATIONS AND CONCLUSION

In this review, a summary was presented on the research examining the influential factors of adolescents' moderate to vigorous physical activity and cardiovascular fitness, including an explanation of the competence motivation theory and a review of its application in pediatric health-related research. The review suggests that there are several influential variables of moderate to vigorous physical activity and health-related fitness in children and adolescents. These factors were further divided by two categories: fixed factors including gender, age, and ethnicity, and flexible factors such as motivational and interpersonal variables. Specifically, the influential factors included: perceived competence, enjoyment, significant others, health status, ethnicity, socioeconomic status, gender, age, and physical education curricula. Interventions aiming to improve moderate to vigorous physical activity and health-related fitness should focus on also improving the aforementioned parameters in order to optimize the odds that a child or adolescent can achieve recommended levels for health and wellbeing.

REFERENCES

Bagoien, T.E., & Halvari, H. (2005). Autonomous motivation: Involvement in physical activity, and perceived sport competence: Structural and mediator models. *Perceptual and Motor Skills, 100*, 3-21.

Barrett, T.M. (2000). *Effects of two cooperative learning strategies on academic learning time, student performance, and social behavior of sixth-grade physical education students* (Unpublished doctoral dissertation). University of Nebraska, Lincoln.

Beauchamp, L., Darst, P.W., & Thompson, L.P. (1990). Academic learning time as an indication of quality high school physical education. *Journal of Physical Education, Recreation and Dance, 61*, 92- 95.

Beckett, K.D. (1989). The effects of motor appropriate engagement ALT-PE (M) on achievement in a badminton skill during an experimental unit. *The Physical Educator, 46*, 36-40.

Bell, K.W. (1997). *The relationship between perceived physical competence and the PA patterns of fifth and seventh grade children* (Unpublished doctoral dissertation). Virginia Polytechnic Institute and State University, Blacksburg.

Birdwell, D. (1980). *The effects of modification of teacher behavior on the academic learning time of selected students in physical education* (Doctoral dissertation). Available from Dissertation Abstracts International. (UMI No. 8022239).

Bois, J.E., Sarrazin, P.G., Brustad, R.J., Trouilloud, D.O., Cury, F. (2005). Elementary schoolchildren are perceived competence and physical activity involvement: The influence of parents' role modeling behaviors and perceptions of their child's competence. *Psychology of Sport and Exercise, 6*, 381-397.

Booth, M., Macaskill, P., Mclellan, L., Phongsavan, P., Okely, T., Patterson, J., et al. (1997). *NSW school fitness and PA survey*. New South Wales, Australia: New South Wales Department of Education and Training.

Borra, S., Schwartz, N., Spain, C., & Natchipolsky, M. (1995). Food, physical activity, and fun: Inspiring America's kids to more healthful lifestyles. *Journal of the American Dietetic Association, 7*, 816-818.

Carroll, B., & Loumidis, L. (2001). Children's perceived competence and enjoyment in physical education and PA outside school. *European Physical Education Review, 7*, 24-43.

Chambers, S. (1991). Factors affecting elementary school student's participation in sports. *The Elementary School Journal, 91*, 413-419.

Craig, S., Goldberg, J., & Dietz, W. (1996). Psychosocial correlates of physical activity among fifth and eighth graders. *Preventive Medicine*, *25*, 506-513.

Crocker, P.R.E., Bouchard, M., & Gessaroli, M.E. (1995). Measuring enjoyment in youth sport setting: A confirmatory factor analysis of the Physical Activity Enjoyment Scale. *Journal of Sport and Exercise Psychology, 17,* 200-205.

De Marco, G.M., Mancini, V.H., Wuest, D.A., & Schempp, P.G. (1996). Becoming reacquainted with once familiar and still valuable tool: Systematic observation methodology revisited. *International Journal of Physical Education, 32*(1), 17-26.

Denham, C., & Lieberman, P. (1980). *Time to learn.* Washington, DC: National Institute of Education.

Digelidis, N., & Papaioannou, A. (1999). Age-group differences in intrinsic motivation, goal orientations and perceptions of athletic competence, physical appearance and motivational climate in Greek physical education. *Scandinavian Journal of Medicine & Science in Sports, 9*, 375–380.

DiLorenzo, T.M., Stucky-Ropp, R.C., VanderWal, J.S., & Gotham, H.J. (1998). Determinants of exercise among children. II. A longitudinal analysis. *Preventive Medicine*, *27*(3), 470-477.

Dodds, P., Rife, F., & Metzler, M. (1982). Academic learning time in physical education: Data collection, completed research and future directions. In M. Pieron & J. Cheffers (Eds), *Studying the teaching in physical education* (37-52). Liege, Belgium: International Association for Physical Education in Higher Education.

Fredricks, J.A., & Eccles, J.S. (2002). Children's competence and value beliefs from childhood through adolescence: Growth trajectories in two male-sex-types domains. *Developmental Psychology, 38*, 519–533.

Fu, Y., Gao, Z., Hannon, J., Shultz, B., Newton, M., & Sibthorp, J. (2013). Influence of a health-related physical fitness model on students' physical activity, perceived competence, and enjoyment. *Perceptual and Motor Skills, 117*(3), 956-970.

Gao, Z. (2008). Perceived competence and enjoyment in predicting students' physical activity levels and cardiorespiratory fitness. *Perceptual and Motor Skills, 107,* 365-372.

Gao, Z. (2009). Students' motivation, engagement, satisfaction, and cardiorespiratory fitness in physical education. *Journal of Applied Sport Psychology, 21*, 102-115.

Gao, Z., Hannon, J.C., Newton, M., & Huang, C. (2011). The effects of curricular activity on students' situational motivation and physical activity levels. *Research Quarterly for Exercise and Sport, 82*, 536-544

Gao, Z., Lee, A.M., Solmon, M.A., & Zhang, T. (2009). Changes in middle school students' motivation toward physical education over one school year. *Journal of Teaching in Physical Education, 28*, 378-399.

Gao, Z., Lodewyk, K., & Zhang, T. (2009). The role of ability beliefs and incentives in middle school students' intentions, cardiovascular fitness, and effort. *Journal of Teaching in Physical Education, 28*, 3-20.

Gao, Z., Newton, M., & Carson, R.L. (2008). Students' motivation, physical activity levels, and health-related physical fitness in fitness class. *Middle Grades Research Journal, 3*(4), 21-39.

Gao, Z., Zhang, P., & Podlog, L. (2013). Examining elementary school children's enjoyment of traditional tag games versus interactive dance games. *Psychology, Health & Medicine,* 1-9.

Gettinger, M. & Seibert, J.K. (2002). Best practices in increasing academic learning time. In A. Thomas & J. Grimes (Ed.), *Best practices in school psychology, 4*(20), 1-16.

Harter, S. (1978). Effectance motivation reconsidered: Toward a developmental model. *Human Development, 1*, 34-64.

Harter, S. (1985). *The self-perception profile for children: Revision of the perceived ccompetence scale for children, manual.* Denver, CO: University of Denver.

Hashim, H., Grove, J.R., & Whipp, P. (2008). Validating the youth sport enjoyment construct in high school physical education. *Research Quarterly for Exercise and Sport, 79,* 183-194.

Hobin, E.P., Leatherdale, S.T., Manske, S., Dubin, J.A., Elliott, S., & Veugelers, P. (2012). A multilevel examination of gender differences in the association between features of the school environment and physical activity among a sample of grades 9 to 12 students in Ontario, Canada. *BMC Public Health, 12*, 74.

Hovell, M. F., Sallis, J. F., Kolody, B., McKenzie, T. L. (1999). Children's physical activity choices: A developmental analysis of gender, intensity levels, and time. *Pediatric Exercise Science, 11*, 158-168.

Jacobs, J.E., Lanza, S., Osgood, D.W., Eccles, J.S., & Wigfield, A. (2002). Changes in children's self-competence and values: Gender and domain differences across grade one through twelve. *Child Development, 73*, 509–527.

Johnson, M.K. (1999). *The effects of classwide peer tutoring in physical education on motor skills and social behaviors of third grade elementary school students* (Unpublished master's thesis). University of Nebraska, Lincoln.

Kalaja, S., Jaakkola, T., Liukkonen, J., & Watt, A. (2010). The role of gender, enjoyment, perceived competence, and fundamental movement skills as correlates of the PA engagement of Finnish physical education students. *Scandinavian Sport Studies Forum, 1*, 69-87.

Kamtsios, S. (2010). Gender differences in elementary school children in perceived athletic competence, body attractiveness, attitudes towards exercise and participation in physical activity. *International Quarterly of Sport Science, 2*, 10-18.

Kremer, J., Trew, K., & Ogle, S. (1997). *Young people's involvement in sport*. London: Routledge.

Lee, A.M. (1996). How the field evolved. In S.J. Silverman & C.D. Ennis (Eds.), *Student learning in physical education. Applying research to enhance instruction* (9-34). Champaign, IL: Human Kinetics.

Martin, J., Kulinna, P.H., McCaughtry, N., Cothran, D., Dake, J., & Fahoome, G. (2005). The theory of planned behavior: Predicting physical activity and cardiorespiratory fitness in African American children. *Journal of Sport and Exercise Psychology, 27*, 456-469.

McKenzie, T. L. (2003). Health-related physical education: Physical activity, fitness, and wellness. In S. T. Silverman & C. D. Ennis (Eds.), *Student learning in physical education: Applying research to enhance instruction* (pp. 207-226). Champaign, IL: Human Kinetics.

McKenzie, T.L., Sallis, J.F., & Rosengard, P. (2009). Beyond the stucco tower: Design, development, and dissemination of the SPARK physical education programs. *Quest, 61*, 114-127.

Metzler, M. (1979). *The measurement of academic learning time in physical education* (Doctoral dissertation). Available from Ohio State University Dissertation and Theses database. (UMI No. 8009314).

Metzler, M. (1989). A review of research on time in sport pedagogy. *Journal of Teaching in Physical Education, 8*, 87-103.

Paese, P.C. (1986). Increasing ALT-PE (M) in the classes of experienced elementary physical education teachers. *Education Clearinghouse.*

Parish, L.E., & Treasure, D.C. (2003). Physical activity and situational motivation in physical education: Influence of the motivational climate and perceived ability. *Research Quarterly for Exercise and Sport, 74*, 173-182.

Placek. J., & Randall. L. (1986). Comparison of academic learning time in physical education: Students of specialists and nonspecialists. *Journal of Teaching in Physical Education, 5*, 157-165.

Prochaska, J.J., Sallis, J.F., Slymen, D.J., & McKenzie, T.L.A. (2003). A longitudinal study of children's enjoyment of physical education. *Pediatric Exercise Science, 15*, 170–178.

Reeve, R.E., & Weiss, M.R. (2006). Sports and physical activities. In George G. Bear & Kathleen M. Minke (Eds.), *Children's needs III: Development, prevention, and intervention* (485-498). Bethesda, MD: National Association for School Psychologists.

Rink, J.E. (1996). Effective instruction in physical education. (In Silverman, & Ennis. 1996). *Student learning in physical education: Applying research to enhance instruction* (171-198). Champaign, IL: Human Kinetics.

Sallis, J.F. (1993). Epidemiology of physical activity and fitness in children and adolescents. *Critical Reviews in Food Science Nutrition. 33*, 405-408.

Sallis, J.F., & Owen, N. (1999). *Physical activity and behavioral medicine.* Thousand Oaks, CA: Sage.

Scanlan, T.K., & Simons, J.P. (1992). The construct of sport enjoyment. In G.C. Roberts (Eds.) *Motivation in sport and exercise* (pp. 199-215). Champaign, IL: Human Kinetics.

Shen, B., McCaughtry, N., & Martin, J. (2007). The influence of self-determination in physical education on leisure-time physical activity behavior. *Research Quarterly for Exercise and Sport, 78*, 328-338.

Shephard, R.J., & Trudeau, F. (2000). The legacy of physical education: Influences on adult lifestyle. *Pediatric Exercise Science, 12*, 34–50.

Siedentop, D. (1983). Academic learning time: Reflections and prospects. *Journal of Teaching in Physical Education, 3*, 3-7.

Siedentop, D., Birdwell, D., & Metzler, M. (1979). A process approach to measuring teaching effectiveness in physical education. Paper presented at the *AAHPERD Convention*, New Orleans.

Silverman, S. (1985). Students' characteristics mediating engagement–outcome relationships in physical education. *Research Quarterly for Exercise and Sport, 56*, 66-72.

Silverman, S., Devillier, R. & Ramirez, T. (1991). The validity of Academic Learning Time-Physical Education (ALT-PE) as a process measure of achievement. *Research Quarterly for Exercise and Sport, 62*(3), 319-325.

Silverman, S., Dodds, P., Placek, J., Shute, S., & Rife, F. (1984). Academic Learning Time in elementary school Physical Education (ALT-PE) for student subgroups and instructional activity units. *Research Quarterly for Exercise and Sport, 55,* 365-370.

Stein, C., Fisher, L., Berkey, C., & Colditz, G. (2007). Adolescent PA and perceived competence: Does change in activity level impact self-perception? *Journal of Adolescent Health, 40,* 462-470.

Telama, R. (1998). Psychological background of a physically active lifestyle among European youth. In R. Naul, K. Hardman, M. Pieron, & B. Skirsted (Eds.), *Physical activity and healthy lifestyles of children and youth* (63-74). Schorndorf: Karl Hofman.

Telama. R., & Yang. X. (2000). Decline of physical activity from youth to young adulthood in Finland. *Medicine and Science in Sports and Exercise, 32,* 1617-1622.

Trost, S.G., Pate, R., Sallis, J., Freedson, P., Taylor, W., Dowda, M., & Sirard, J. (2002). Age and gender differences in objectively measured physical activity in youth. *Medicine and Science in Sports and Exercise, 34*, 350-355.

U. S Department of Health and Human Services. (1996). *PA and health: A report of the Surgeon General.* Atlanta, Ga: US Dept of Health and Human Services, Centers for Disease Control and Prevention; 1996.

Wallhead, T.L., & Buckworth, J. (2004). The role of physical education in the promotion of youth physical activity. *Quest, 56*, 285-301.

Wankel, L.M. (1993). The importance of enjoyment to adherence and psychological benefits from physical activity. *International Journal of Sport Psychology, 24*, 151-169.

Wankel, L.M. (1997). "Strawpersons," selective reporting and inconsistent logic: A response to Kimiecik and Harris's analysis of enjoyment. *Journal of Sport and Exercise Psychology, 19*, 98-109.

Weiss, M.R., & Williams, L. (2004). The why of youth sport involvement: A development perspective on motivational process. In M. R. Weiss (Ed.), *Developmental sport and exercise psychology: A lifespan perspective* (223-268). Morgantown, WV: Fitness Information Technology.

Whaley, G.M. (1980). *The effect of daily monitoring and feedback to teachers and students on academic learning time-physical education* (Doctoral dissertation). Available from Dissertation Abstract International. (UMI No.8022365).

Williams, L., & Gill, D. (1995). The role of perceived competence in the motivation of physical activity. *Journal of Sport & Exercise Psychology, 17,* 363-378.

Yli-Piipari, S., Watt, A., Jaakkola, T., Liukkonen, J., & Nurmi, J. (2009). Relationships between physical education students' motivational profiles, enjoyment, state anxiety, and self-reported physical activity. *Journal of Sports Science and Medicine, 8,* 327-336.

Editors' Contact Information

Dr. Zan Gao
School of Kinesiology, the University of Minnesota
207 Cooke Hall, 1900 University Ave. SE
Minneapolis, MN 55455
Email: gaoz@umn.edu

Zachary Pope
Masters of Kinesiology
School of Kinesiology, University of Minnesota
1900 University Ave. SE
Minneapolis, MN 55455
Email: popex157@umn.edu

INDEX

D

E

J

K

L

M

N

O

P

R

S

T

U

V

W

Y